Praise for Isa Chandra Moskowitz's *Veganomicon*

"This is vegan cooking at its best." —*Vegetarian Times*

"Exuberant and unapologetic … Moskowitz and Romero's recipes don't skimp on fat or flavor, and the eclectic collection of dishes is a testament to the authors' sincere love of cooking and culinary exploration." —*Saveur*

"[T]his slam-bang effort from vegan chefs Moskowitz and Romero (*Vegan with a Vengeance*) is thorough and robust, making admirable use of every fruit and vegetable under the sun." —*Publishers Weekly* starred review

"Full of recipes for which even a carnivore would give up a night of meat."
—*San Francisco Chronicle*

"The next revolution in neo-vegan cuisine." —*Philadelphia City Paper*

"Spending time with [Moskowitz's] cheerfully politicized book feels like hanging out with Grace Paley. She and her cooking partner, Terry Hope Romero, are as crude and funny when kibbitzing as they are subtle and intuitive when putting together vegan dishes that are full of non-soggy adult tastes." —*New York Times Book Review*

"For those of us whose definition of 'vegan' includes a love-of-cooking clause, this book is exactly what its subhead claims: the ultimate." —*VegNews*

"It's full of great food that anyone would love." —*Baltimore Sun*

"User-friendly, packed with tips and instructions for a wide range of cooking techniques." —*New York Sun*

"Veganomicon is perfect for the beginner vegan chef." —*News & Observer*

"Even carnivorous diners won't miss the meat." —*Winston-Salem Journal*

"I highly recommend this book to all cooks, but if you're shopping for a vegan or vegetarian friend, this book is a must." —*Herald-Times*

"The *Betty Crocker's Cookbook* of the vegan world." —*Bitch*

"[A] witty book that's great for cooks." —*Fresno Bee*

"Seriously good recipes with broad appeal." —*Washington Post*

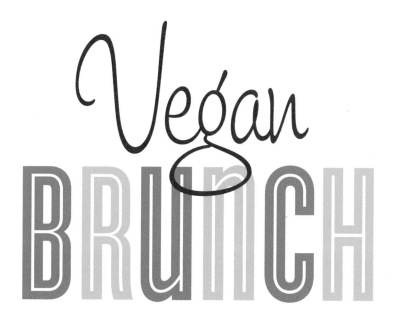

Vegan BRUNCH

ALSO BY ISA CHANDRA MOSKOWITZ

Veganomicon

Vegan Cupcakes Take Over the World

Vegan with a Vengeance

Vegan BRUNCH

Homestyle Recipes

Worth Waking Up For— from Asparagus Omelets to Pumpkin Pancakes

Isa Chandra Moskowitz

Da Capo

LIFE LONG

A Member of the Perseus Books Group

Design by Jane Raese
Set in 10-point ITC Century

Cataloging-in-Publication Data for this book is available from the Library of Congress.

First Da Capo Press edition 2009
ISBN 978-0-7382-1272-2

Published by Da Capo Press
A Member of the Perseus Books Group
www.dacapopress.com

Da Capo Press books are available at special discounts for bulk purchases in the U.S. by corporations, institutions, and other organizations. For more information, please contact the Special Markets Department at the Perseus Books Group, 2300 Chestnut Street, Suite 200, Philadelphia, PA, 19103, or call (800) 810-4145, ext. 5000, or e-mail special.markets@ perseusbooks.com.

10 9 8 7 6 5 4 3

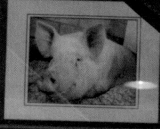

Dedicated to
vegan hash slingers
everywhere.
Scrambled tofu
saves lives!

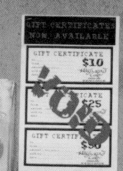

Why Vegan?

meet your
meat

SEVEN

SEVEN

Contents

The Savory

Scrambles, Omelets, and Skillet Favorites You'll Devour

The Sweet

Pancakes, Waffles, French Toast, and
Anything That Will Have You Licking Syrup from Your Plate

The Sides

Potatoes, Sausages, and a Stuffed Veggie or Two—
Everything You Need to Make Brunch Complete

The Bread Basket

Scrumptiousness from the Oven, from Muffins to Bagels

The Toppings

Gravy, Sauces, and Spreads to Mess Up Your Bib

The Drinks

Just When You Thought You Knew How to Make a Smoothie

Introduction

Welcome to *Vegan Brunch!* Put on your fluffiest slippers, slip on that thrift store apron, and pour yourself a hot cup of coffee. Let's get started.

Skeptics accuse brunch of being nothing but a glorified breakfast. Well, yeah, kinda. But breakfast in this day and age is just a muffin in one hand, a mad rush to work, and crumbs all over your shirt. Breakfast is whatever we eat first thing in the morning, but brunch is an event. More than any other meal, brunch seems to have a purpose in our lives that isn't just about the food being served. It's a time to catch up with friends. Time to slow down. Time to hatch great plans, to get all hyped up on coffee, and say dumb stuff that haunts you for the rest of your life.

Brunch is also hands down the best meal to host. You can serve seasonal creations for any occasion. From coffee to cinnamon, the aromas of brunch are always so warm and alluring, so downright cozy and homey, there is just no going wrong. Whether it's a crowded, shoulder-to-shoulder event with ten of your best friends, a way to tell your family that you love them more than instant oatmeal can say, or an intimate time to flip omelets with a pal (or a crush), brunch is the best time to break out the e-vites and warm up your oven mitts.

The typical cravings I get for brunch are usually smoky and earthy and herby: fennel, mushroom, sage, thyme, tempeh. But the biggest question is always, savory or sweet? My favorite way to decide is "both." As in a big plate of scrambled tofu, but also a plate of syrup-drenched pancakes for everyone to split. In the winter, you can top pancakes with cinnamon apples; in the summer, with blueberries and lemon.

Within these pages you'll find recipes to suit your every desire. Many of the recipes will be familiar to anyone who's ever stepped foot into an American diner, only veganized. There are omelets made with pureed tofu, French toast dipped in pumpkin, tempeh-based crab cakes. I love to replicate traditional

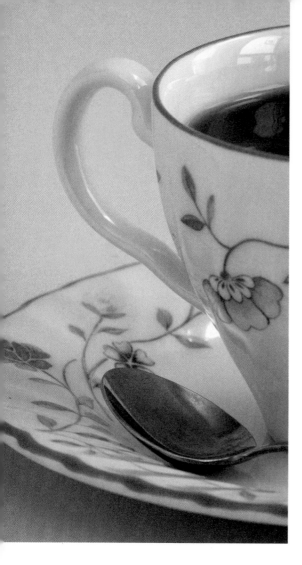

dishes for special occasions—first of all, because it's fun, and second of all, because it creates food choices that are better for the animals, better for the planet, and better for you. Other recipes were inspired by food from around the world, also known as anything you can eat for brunch in New York City. That includes spicy Indian dosas and Polish pierogi smothered in caramelized onions.

I wrote this book in hopes that it would inspire you to call up some friends and bond over a plate of potatoes. I've had so much fun making the recipes for my own loved ones and I hope that you will, too. Nothing is as delicious as a day off, good music playing, warm food for your belly, and the knowledge that you did it all without harming any of our fluffy friends.

With love from Portland,
Isa

The Vegan Brunch Pantry

This is not an exhaustive list of every pantry item you might need, just a list of ingredients that appear in many recipes. I did try to make the recipes as pantry-friendly as possible, but brunch is a great reason to pick up a few specialty items.

NUTRITIONAL YEAST

Sometimes called "nooch," sometimes called vegan fairy dust, nutritional yeast lends a cheesy flavor to sauces and scrambles. Available in flakes or powder form, nutritional yeast is usually found in the bulk bins of your health food store. It's also available in plastic jars, but make sure that the brand you choose is vegan, as some manufacturers list the inexplicable addition of whey. I store my nooch in the fridge. Nutritional yeast is nothing like brewer's yeast or any other kind of yeast, so don't go replacing it. A popular brand is Red Star.

CORNMEAL

I do so love the sunny, shiny taste and crunchy texture that cornmeal lends to baked goods, pancakes, and waffles. Purchase at most supermarkets in boxes or bags and often in bulk. The recipes in this book were developed with medium-ground cornmeal, but fine-ground will work, too, just a little less crunchy.

CHICKPEA FLOUR

Chickpea flour is just what the name implies—ground up, lightly roasted chickpeas. It lends an eggy flavor to omelets and crepes as well as a pretty, pale yellow color. To top it off, it provides a fluffy texture, so hey, thanks for everything, chickpea flour! Purchase at Indian markets, where it's called *besan*, or at Middle Eastern or Israeli markets. It's also available in bulk at your supermarket or health food store or in plastic bags from Bob's Red Mill. Store chickpea flour in your pantry in a tightly sealed container or in your fridge.

CASHEWS

From sauces to quiche, this creamy nut seems to sneak its way into everything. To save money, purchase cashew pieces instead of whole cashews. The recipes were developed with unroasted and unsalted, but I've been known to wash the salt off a roasted cashew in my day. Buy them in the bulk section of your supermarket or in big bags at Trader Joe's. Store cashews in the freezer for maximum freshness.

VITAL WHEAT GLUTEN

Nothing beats VWG for making chewy scrumptious fake meats that hold together and don't have a health food-y taste. VWG is the pure protein of wheat, available in a convenient flour form for your purchasing pleasure. Two brands that I recommend are Arrowhead Mills and Bob's Red Mill. You may have to go to a health food store to find it, but sometimes it is available in everyday supermarkets in the baking section.

BLACK SALT (*KALA NAMAK*)

Black salt is actually pink, which can be a little confusing. Black salt has a distinctive sulfuric taste akin to egg yolks, so I use it in eggy recipes, like the omelets. There are other kinds of black salt so make sure that you are purchasing Indian black salt, also called *kala namak*. A little goes a long way, so purchase in small amounts if you can. It's available in Indian grocery stores at much more reasonable prices than at a specialty salt shop. The recipes in this book were developed with fine-ground.

SMOKED SALT

While Tofu Benny is the only recipe that calls for smoked salt, I'm going to put it here anyway because you can sprinkle it over anything and everything— potatoes, scrambled tofu or tempeh ... maybe not pancakes, but who knows? There are many varieties of smoked salt, but my two favorites are applewood and hickory. That just refers to the kind of wood used to smoke it.

LIQUID SMOKE

If you crave smokiness in the morning then this is the stuff for you. Liquid smoke is exactly that, smoke from smoldering wood that has been condensed into its liquid form. I'm not going to explain the entire science of it, as I would like you to stay awake to enjoy your brunch, but rest assured that it is vegan, it is natural, and it isn't anything you should be scared of. Embrace liquid smoke. It's available in the condiment section of your supermarket.

TOFU, ALL TYPES

Would you dream of having just one pair of legwarmers? No, you have a pair for a casual stroll down the beach, a pair for an elegant ballroom evening, a pair for high-powered business meetings, and so on. So should you have many types of tofu. Some situations call for silken, some for extra-firm, some for soft. Read through the recipes carefully and use the type of tofu suggested or don't come complaining to me.

TEMPEH

When you call tempeh a fermented soybean cake it doesn't sound all that great. But when prepared correctly, tempeh is a succulent, toothsome addition to your brunch table. It's become increasingly available in supermarkets, but you may have to make a health food store trip for your 'peh.

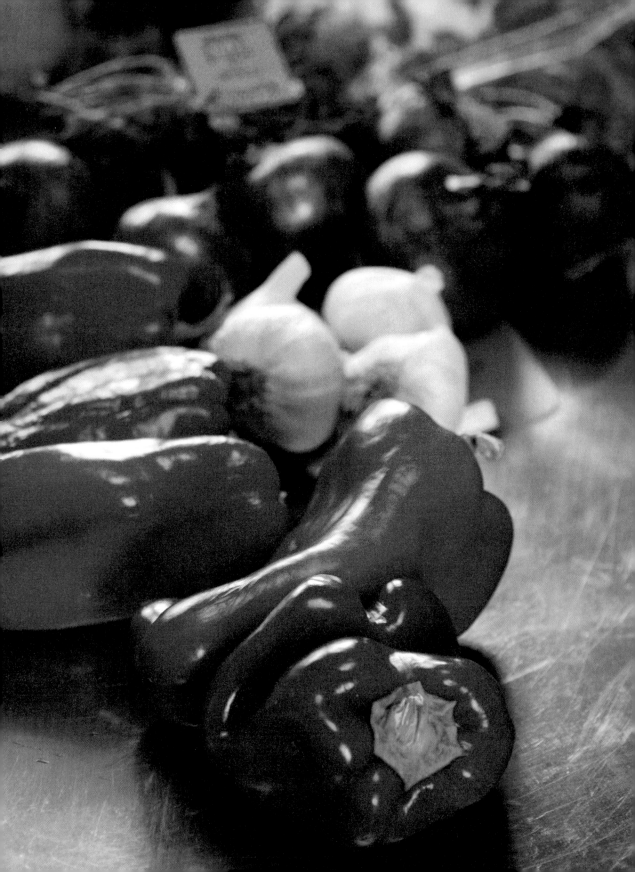

Setting Up and Serving Up Brunch in Style

PLAN YOUR MENU

There are plenty of pairing suggestions for recipes throughout this book, but I have a few general thoughts for menu planning.

My main entertaining tip is this: don't overextend yourself. In all honesty, this book could just be scrambled tofu, roasted potatoes, and pancakes. You might feel ripped off, but your guests would be satisfied. Of course, that is not to say don't try out new things, just that brunch shouldn't be too stressful. You want to be able to enjoy yourself as well. If you are just joining the world of brunch hosting then build up your repertoire. Start with the easy recipes, like any of the scrambles or French toasts, and then move on to more ambitious dishes, like omelets and crepes. Rest assured that all of these recipes have been tested by our trusty team of recipe warriors and are guaranteed to be as foolproof as possible.

When entertaining, it's a good idea to cook at least one dish you are comfortable with and ideally have made before. If this is your first time with waffles or omelets, give them a test run for dinner sometime during the week. Make sure to read all of your recipes all the way through so that you don't miss any steps. If something needs to sit in the fridge for an hour or to marinate, you don't want to be surprised! Don't let that scare you, though—I will include a note in the recipe intro if that is the case.

There's nothing like the aroma of brewing coffee mingling with the steamy sounds of hair metal. But maybe hair metal isn't your thing. Even if you aren't into Faster Pussycat, play some music in your kitchen that gets you going. Turn it up loud before your guests arrive, have fun, do stupid dances, cook in a bra and panties—even if you're a guy.

MISE EN PLACE

There's a movie with this quote: "*Mise en place*—that's French for everything in its effing place!" Basically, it is. Before you start cooking, have not just all your ingredients, but any measuring cup, mixing bowl, and pot or pan you might need ready and waiting. It will save you so much time and heartache in the long run: take five minutes or so to set yourself up.

CREATE A COFFEE STATION

Brunch without coffee is like swimming with no water. Any apparatus will do; French press, percolator, Melitta filter, gigantic, someone-just-died coffee urn. You don't need anything fancy.

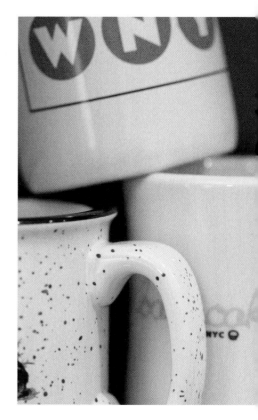

No matter the size of your pad, you can set up an easily accessible coffee station to keep your guests fueled throughout brunch. Find a nice, quiet corner. If there isn't already an un-cluttered surface available, then move a side table on in. Set up your coffee maker and put out mugs, spoons, sugars and creamer, and anything else guests might want for coffee. A cinnamon sprinkler? Some raspberry coffee syrup? Sure, why not. You might want to pregrind some coffee, too—that way you're never far away from your next brew.

SERVING AND PLATING

Deciding whether to plate the food or have guests serve themselves is probably the biggest decision a brunch host will have to make, right above "Do I splurge on the soy creamer?" There are serving suggestions throughout the book for individual recipes, but I have a few rules of thumb.

If there are six or fewer guests, I plate for them. I do this because it's fun to feel like a real chef, garnishes and all, but also because I will have a clearer idea of what portion sizes should be than my guests will. One person might create a potato mountain, leaving only a tiny piece of onion for someone else to push back and forth across their plate.

If you aren't worried about potato misappropriation, then setting the food out family style is great, too, so long as you have enough serving plates. Don't have guests in the kitchen serving themselves off the stove. Have some class and transfer that scrambled tofu to a serving bowl. And don't forget the serving spoon! A big tablespoon works fine, just make sure there is a utensil for each dish so that people aren't using their own forks to serve themselves.

You can also mix and match serving styles, plating some dishes but leaving some out on the table as well. You can also ignore me completely and just do whatever makes the most sense for your menu.

SEATING

Unless you have a banquet table in your *maison*, you may be short on seating. If your guests outnumber your seats at the table, then scrap the table, just use it to serve food. Move all the chairs out to a common area, ideally by the couch. If there still isn't enough seating, throw some pillows onto the floor and utilize whatever sturdy furniture you can—coffee tables, side tables, kitchen stools. You don't have to have an official chair for everyone, but make sure you create a few comfy spots for the seatless. I prefer this floor plan to the one where some people are sitting at the table and some are sitting in another room on a floor. That can be okay, and I suppose it's just personal preference, but I feel like it creates this disparity between table guests and non-table guests. The last thing you need is a floor guest uprising that leaves your brunch in shambles.

Silverware

Put all the silverware in a container or cup in the middle of the table. Really, it's just forks. You don't usually need a knife with vegan food, we're just nonviolent like that.

Glasses

Ideally you'll have a water glass and then another glass for juice or mimosas. But don't sweat it if guests need to alternate between a water and juice. Whatever prevents you from buying disposable cups is what you gotta do. Keep glasses on the table beside the plates.

Drinks

If your table isn't large enough, then use a little side table to keep drinks within arm's reach. A folding tray would work great here. It's nice to have pitchers for juices, but it's often easier to slum it with a carton of OJ right there in plain sight. Save the pitchers for sangria.

Napkins

Cloth napkins seem like an extravagance, but beautiful linen ones are often available in thrift stores for pennies. Not only are they better for the environment, but they're easier on the wallet, too. But what do I know? I don't even have a wallet.

Condiments: Jams, Jellies, Butters, Syrups, Sauces, etc.

Place jellies on the table with a spoon for each of them. Even if you aren't serving pancakes or sweet dishes, it's nice to serve jellies and jams for toast to satisfy that morning sugar craving. Keep spreads like vegan butter, cream cheese, and/or homemade spreads on the table with their own butter knives or spreaders. Serve maple syrup in a small gravy boat or pitcher. That stuff is expensive and a smaller container will make guests less eager to bathe their food in it. Since people like to ruin everything with ketchup, I suppose you can put some of that out, too. And don't forget the hot sauce!

The Savory

Scrambles, Omelets,
and Skillet Favorites
You'll Devour

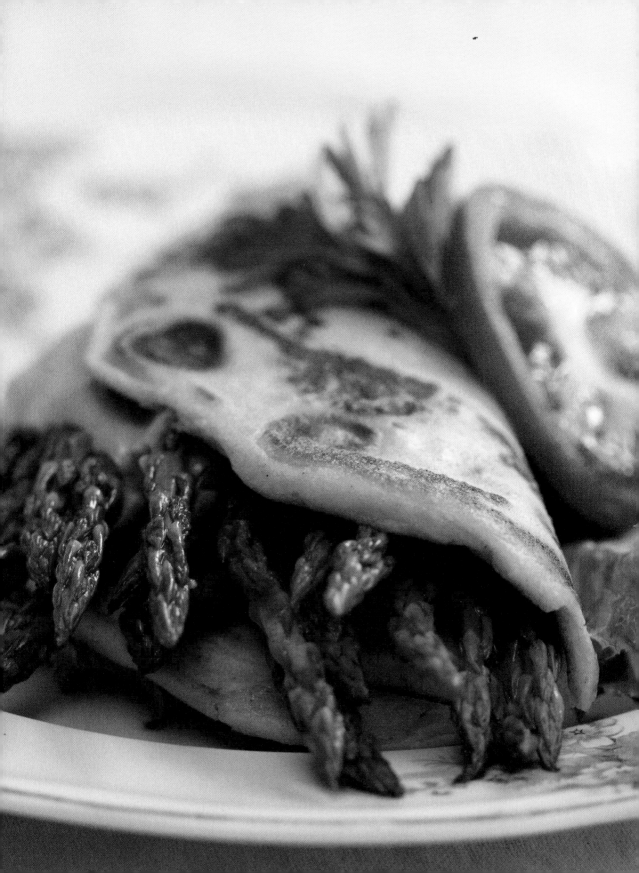

Tofu Omelets

Makes 4 omelets

There's something about an omelet that says, It's the weekend, dig in! Get ready for a day that's all your own! But what to expect from a tofu omelet? Not an exact replica of an egg omelet, but delicious nonetheless. Chickpea flour gives the tofu fluffiness and an egglike taste. Nutritional yeast adds color as well as delectable savory flavor. Turmeric goes the rest of the way for that sunshine yellow hue. And then … black salt. If you haven't tried it before, and you love the taste of eggs, you are in for a real treat. This Indian salt, also called *kala namak*, has a sulfuric taste that is reminiscent of egg yolks. I like to add some to the omelet batter and also sprinkle it on at the end for an even stronger taste. However, if you are averse to the taste of eggs, you may skip this and just use ¾ teaspoon of regular sea salt in the omelet.

2 garlic cloves (optional)

1 pound silken tofu, lightly drained (not the vacuum-packed kind) or soft tofu (see tip on page 14); Nasoya brand is recommended

2 tablespoons nutritional yeast

2 tablespoons olive oil

½ teaspoon turmeric

1 teaspoon fine black salt, plus extra for sprinkling (optional, see note to the left)

½ cup chickpea flour

1 tablespoon arrowroot or cornstarch

Chop up the garlic, if using, in a food processor. Add the tofu, nutritional yeast, olive oil, turmeric, and salt. Puree until smooth. Add the chickpea flour and arrowroot and puree again for about 10 seconds, until combined. Make sure to scrape down the sides so that everything is well incorporated.

Preheat a large, heavy-bottomed, nonstick skillet over medium-high heat. Well-seasoned cast iron works great or use a regular nonstick skillet. Lightly grease the pan with either cooking spray or a very thin layer of oil. (The less oil the better for the nice brown speckles we're going for.) Also, make sure that you use a large skillet, as you need room to spread out the omelet and to get your spatula under there to flip. Don't use an 8-inch omelet pan or anything like that. Here you'll need at least 12 inches (tee hee).

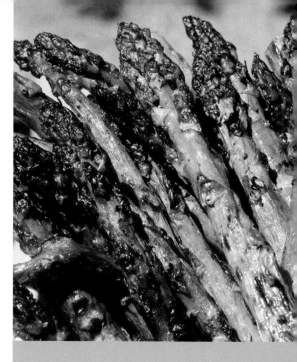

In ½-cup increments, pour the omelet batter into the skillet. Use the back of a spoon or a rubber spatula to spread the batter out into about 6-inch circles. (It's okay if it isn't a perfect circle.) Be gentle—if there are any rips or holes, that is fine, just gently fill them in as you spread the batter.

Let the batter cook for about 3 to 5 minutes before flipping. The top of the omelet should dry and become a matte yellow when it's ready to be flipped. If you try and it seems like it might fall apart, give it a little more time. When the omelet is ready to be flipped, the underside should be flecked light to dark brown. Flip the omelet and cook for about a minute on the other side. Keep warm on a plate covered with tinfoil as you make the remaining omelets.

Fill omelet with the filling of your choice (page 15), then fold it. Once the omelet has been filled, sprinkle with a little extra black salt, since some of its flavor disappears when cooked.

TIP If using soft tofu, some trial and error may be required because the water content varies so drastically from brand to brand. Some of my recipe testers added up to ½ cup of water and it worked beautifully. But if you're going to experiment, and you should, do so in half batches and try to have fun with it. (For example, don't do it when you have company coming over and don't do it if you're PMS-ing and apt to throw a blenderful of pureed tofu at the wall.)

I find it's best to start by adding ¼ cup of water to the batter. Do a mini omelet test by pouring 2 tablespoons into the pan. If the batter spreads out on its own and firms up when cooking, then you are good to go. If it just sits there in a mound and doesn't move, then add up to ¼ cup more water to the batter.

✵ VARIATIONS ✵

Fillings:
It's What's Inside That Counts

It's hard for me to imagine produce that wouldn't find its calling stuffed into an omelet. When it comes to omelet fillings, think fresh and you can't go wrong. Look deep within yourself that morning and find your spirit vegetable. If that doesn't do it for you, hit up your farmers' market and go with what's in season. Each of these fillings makes enough for four omelets. Mix and match them to your heart's content and come up with scrumptious fillings of your own.

MUSHROOMS AND SPINACH

Preheat a large pan over medium heat. Sauté **4 cups sliced cremini mushrooms** in **2 tablespoons olive oil.** After about 5 minutes, when mushrooms are soft, add **2 minced garlic cloves** and about **3 tablespoons chopped fresh thyme.** Sauté about 3 minutes more, add **fresh black pepper** and a few dashes of **salt** to taste. Stuff into omelets and divide **2 cups of chopped fresh spinach** among them. The spinach will wilt in the omelet. Top with Cheesy Sauce (page 217) or **shredded vegan cheese** and fold.

GRILLED MARINATED ASPARAGUS

Marinate **1 pound asparagus,** ends trimmed, in a mixture of ¼ **cup balsamic vinegar, ¼ cup olive oil, 2 smashed garlic cloves, fresh black pepper,** and a generous pinch of **salt.** Let sit for at least an hour or overnight. Grill asparagus on a preheated hot grill or grill pan for about 8 minutes, flipping once. Divide among omelets, top with Miso Tahini Sauce (page 220), and fold.

ROASTED TOMATOES, RICOTTA, AND BASIL

Preheat the oven to 300°F. Slice **2 pounds plum tomatoes** lengthwise. Toss with **2 tablespoons olive oil.** Sprinkle with **salt** and **fresh black pepper.** Place tomatoes face down on a rimmed baking sheet and roast for about an hour and a half. Stuff omelet with Cashew Ricotta (page 219) and about **10 leaves fresh basil** for each, then add tomatoes and fold.

SAUSAGE AND PEPPERS

Preheat a large pan over medium-high heat. Sauté four Sausages (page 137) and **2 medium diced red bell peppers** in **2 tablespoons olive oil.** Stuff into omelets and, if you like, top with Cheesy Sauce (page 217) or **shredded vegan cheese** and fold.

SHREDDED SWISS CHARD

Use **one bunch of chard**. Remove stems and layer leaves on top of each other. Roll lengthwise into a bundle and thinly slice. Preheat a large pan over medium heat. Sauté **3 minced garlic cloves** in **2 tablespoons olive oil** for about 2 minutes. Add chard and sauté until completely wilted, adding splashes of water if necessary to get it to cook down. **Salt** to taste. Stuff into omelets and top with Cheesy Sauce (page 217) or sprinkle with **shredded vegan cheese** and fold.

BURNT BROCCOLI

My aunt Bonnie invented burnt broccoli, probably by accident. It's simple and even a little silly, but I absolutely love it. Preheat a large pan over medium heat. Sauté **4 cups broccoli florets** in **2 tablespoons olive oil**. Leave them alone for 2 minutes at a time so they can get a bit charred, then flip. Do this for about 15 minutes. Sprinkle on **salt** to taste. Stuff into omelets and sprinkle with shredded **vegan cheese** if you like, and fold.

OMELET RANCHEROS

Use the bean recipe from Polenta Rancheros (page 51) to stuff into omelets. Top with fresh salsa and Guacamole (page 221).

CAPERS AND BROCCOLI RABE

This is a favorite, and maybe the only combination where vegan cheese is a requirement for me. Preheat a large pan over medium heat. Sauté **3 minced garlic cloves** in **2 tablespoons olive oil**. Add **1 bunch of chopped broc-**

coli rabe. Sauté for about 7 minutes. Add **2 tablespoons capers** and sauté just until heated through. Divide among omelets, top with **shredded vegan cheese,** and serve.

GUACAMOLE AND POTATO

1 recipe Guacamole (page 221), **½ recipe** Diner Home Fries (page 117). Serve salad on the side instead of potatoes.

TEMPEH BACON AND CARAMELIZED ONION

Divide a **½ recipe** Tempeh Bacon Revamped (page 141) and **1 recipe of the caramelized onions** in the Caramelized Vidalia Onion Quiche (page 43) into omelets and fold.

DENVER OMELET

Preheat a large pan over medium heat. Sauté **1½ cups diced seitan, 1 diced small red onion,** and **1 diced green pepper** in **2 tablespoons olive oil** for about 10 minutes, or until browned. Drizzle in **½ teaspoon liquid smoke** and cook for a minute more. Stuff filling into omelets, sprinkle on **vegan cheese** if you like, and fold.

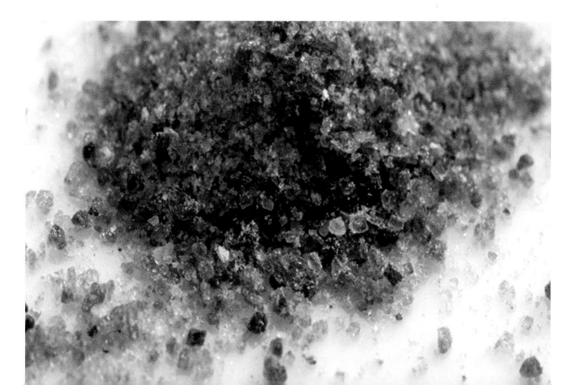

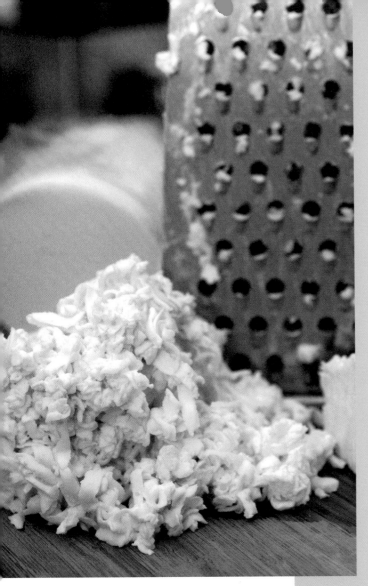

"Cheeze," It Is a-Changin'

Many years ago I never would have suggested we use vegan cheese for anything but feeding to our enemies. But things have changed a lot and I do enjoy using vegan cheese every now and again. There are two brands in particular that I recommend because they do actually melt and they taste pretty good, to boot. Both are available via mail order from Food Fight! Vegan Grocery (www.foodfightgrocery.com).

Teese comes from our good friends at Chicago Soydairy and is available in cute red plastic tubes. I recommend the mozzarella; it has a nice, mellow, tangy flavor and a silky texture when melted.

Cheezly is imported from the United Kingdom and has a range of different flavors from gouda to cheddar, but the one I recommend is the mozzarella "super-melting" style. It has a sharper flavor than Teese but doesn't melt quite as well.

To get your vegan cheese to melt, always shred it, never slice. Once folded into the omelet you can place the omelet back in the pan, over low heat, and cover the pan. Check in about 2 minutes, but it could take up to 5 for the cheese to fully melt. Just take care that the heat is low so that you don't burn your perfect omelet.

Basic Scrambled Tofu

Serves 4

Scrambled tofu is probably what springs to mind when you think of vegan brunch. And if you're going by the countless restaurant menus across America, it might just be the only thing to eat for vegan brunch! I've had one too many disappointing scrambles in my day. Infractions ranged from flavorless heaps of greasy mush to way overspiced, grainy disasters. As simple a concept as it is, some people just don't get scrambled tofu.

For me, a basic scramble should have nice big tofu pieces in it. It's crumbled, yes, but not completely in crumbles. Just kind of torn apart and then broken up a bit when cooking in the pan. The flavor should be lip-smacking and just a bit salty, but not overly so. You shouldn't feel like you are sampling every single item in the spice rack. Garlic, some cumin, a little thyme—that is the base. From there, you can come up with countless variations using whatever is in your fridge that morning.

So this is my basic recipe. There are several more daring plays on scrambled tofu to follow, but when you want a trustworthy and easy-to-modify standard scramble, this makes a great go-to.

For the spice blend:

2 teaspoons ground cumin

1 teaspoon dried thyme, crushed with your fingers

½ teaspoon ground turmeric

1 teaspoon salt

3 tablespoons water

For the tofu:

3 garlic cloves, minced (or more, to taste)

2 tablespoons olive oil

1 pound extra-firm tofu, drained

¼ cup nutritional yeast

Fresh black pepper, to taste

First blend the spices and salt together in a small cup. Add the water and mix. Set aside.

Preheat a large, heavy-bottomed pan over medium-high heat. Sauté the garlic in olive oil for about a minute. Break the tofu apart into bite-size pieces and sauté for about 10 minutes, stirring often. Get under the tofu when you are stirring, scrape

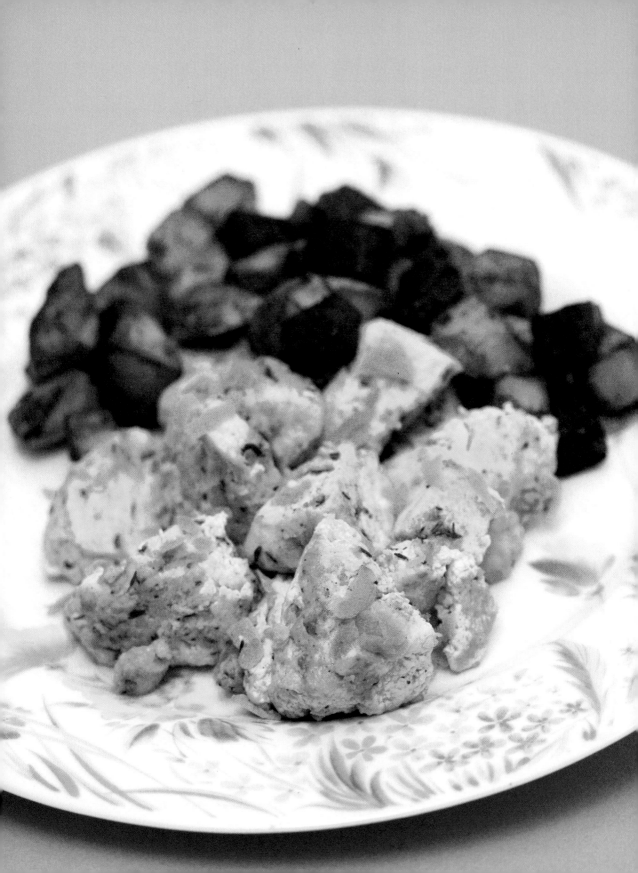

the bottom, and don't let it stick to the pan; that is where the good, crispy stuff is. (Use a thin metal spatula to get the job done; a wooden or plastic one won't really cut it.) The tofu should brown on at least one side, but you don't need to be too precise about it. The water should cook out of it and not collect too much at the bottom of the pan. If that is happening, turn the heat up and let the water evaporate. Conversely, if the scramble seems dry add splashes of water until it's nice and moist.

Add the spice blend and mix to incorporate. Add the nutritional yeast and pepper. Cook for about 5 more minutes. Serve warm.

※ VARIATIONS ※

Tof-u and Tof-me: Scramble Add-Ins

You can include these additions to your scramble by themselves or in combination with one another.

BROCCOLI

Cut **broccoli** into about **1 cup** of small florets and thinly sliced stems. Add along with the tofu.

ONION

Finely chop **1 small onion**. Add along with the garlic and cook for about 5 minutes, until translucent. Proceed with recipe.

RED BELL PEPPERS

Remove stem and seeds and finely chop **1 red bell pepper**. Add along with the garlic and cook for about 5 minutes. Proceed with recipe.

MUSHROOMS

Thinly slice about **1 cup mushrooms**. Add along with the tofu.

OLIVES

Chop about ⅓ **cup sliced olives**. Add towards the end of cooking, after mixing in the nutritional yeast. I love to use black olives, but use whatever you like.

SPINACH

Add about **1 cup chopped spinach** towards the end of cooking, after mixing in the nutritional yeast. Cook until completely wilted.

CARROTS

Grate ½ **an average-size carrot** into the scramble towards the end of cooking. This is a great way to add color to the scramble.

AVOCADO

I almost always have **avocado** with my scramble. Just peel, slice, and serve on top.

Cabbage Patch Tip

Slicing the cabbage for this recipe (page 23) is really easy and a great way to slice cabbage in general. Cut it in half from stem to bottom. Reserve one half for some other use. Now slice your half in half from stem to bottom again, and slice each of those halves across in ¼-inch slices or so.

Curry Scrambled Tofu with Cabbage and Caraway

Serves 4

This scramble was inspired by my middle name, Chandra, being Indian and my last name, Moskowitz, being Russian. I like to think I have imaginary ancestors who migrated from Siberia into China to pick up some tofu, then down into India for spices, even though they already had some caraway in their pocket. Oh, also, they were vegan. Serve with Red Flannel Hash (page 119) to keep going with the Russian theme or Samosa Mashed Potato Pancakes (page 125) to go with the Indian theme.

2 tablespoons olive oil

1 medium red onion, thinly sliced

2 teaspoons caraway seeds

3 to 4 garlic cloves, minced

1 pound extra-firm tofu, cubed

2 to 3 teaspoons curry powder

½ teaspoon ground cumin

¾ teaspoon salt

½ small head red cabbage, thinly sliced (see tip on page 22)

Preheat a large, heavy-bottomed pan over medium-high heat. Sauté onion and caraway seeds in oil for 5 to 7 minutes. Add garlic and sauté for another 30 seconds or so. Add tofu and cook for about 10 minutes, stirring often, until tofu has browned on some of the sides. Add curry powder, cumin, and salt and some splashes of water if the tofu seems too dry. Mix in the cabbage. Cover and cook for 8 to 10 minutes, stirring occasionally, until cabbage is wilted and tender. Taste for spice and add another teaspoon of curry powder if needed (it will depend on the strength of your curry powder).

Basic Scrambled Tempeh

Serves 4

I absolutely adore the succulent, grainy, earthy, nutty flavor of tempeh for brunch, especially during the fall and winter months. Here it's sautéed with some dark, leafy greens and snappy red peppers. I keep the seasoning to a minimum here—a little thyme, fresh black pepper, and salt let the flavors of the tempeh and veggies shine through. I really love to pair earthy with sweet, so Roasted Butternut Squash (page 148) makes a great side.

Preheat a large, heavy-bottomed pan (preferably cast iron) over medium heat. Sauté the tempeh in 2 tablespoons olive oil for about 7 minutes, stirring often, until lightly browned. Add red bell pepper and onion and drizzle in remaining tablespoon of oil. Sauté for about 5 minutes; veggies should be softened but still have a bit of crunch. Add garlic and thyme, sauté for 2 minutes more. Season with salt and pepper. Add Swiss chard and sauté just until wilted. Serve immediately.

3 tablespoons olive oil, divided

1 pound tempeh, cubed

1 red bell pepper, thinly sliced

1 small red onion, thinly sliced (about ½ a cup)

3 garlic cloves, minced

2 teaspoons dried thyme, or 2 tablespoons chopped fresh thyme

¼ teaspoon salt

Fresh black pepper

4 large leaves Swiss chard, or any leafy green, torn into pieces

TIP Some people prefer to steam the tempeh before cooking for a juicier texture. It also reduces the bitterness of the tempeh. I happen to like this dish as is, but if you usually find that tempeh is a bit too bitter for your taste, cube the tempeh and steam for 10 minutes, then proceed with the recipe.

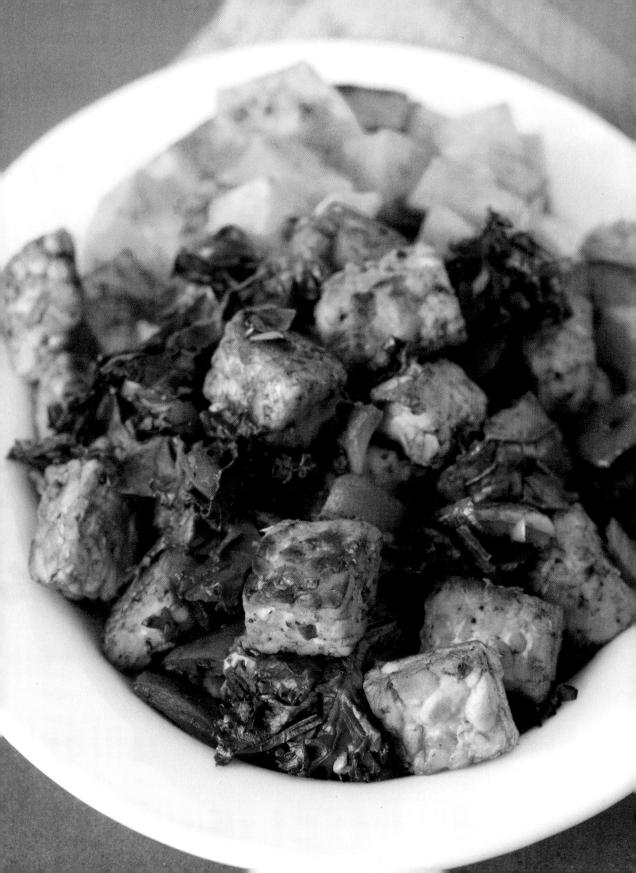

Pesto Scrambled Tofu with Grape Tomatoes

Serves 2 to 4

Pesto—not just for dinner anymore. Luscious basil, juicy cherry tomatoes, and sweet red onions make this a sultry dish, perfect for the morning after. After what? Uh, rearranging your sock drawer? Filing your taxes?

Make ahead: You can make the pesto the night before and keep in the fridge in a tightly sealed container.

As the name suggests, pine nuts, also called pignolis, are actually the seed of pinecones from several specific species of pine tree. Keep your pine nuts in the freezer to prevent them from going rancid. Toast them straight from the freezer as needed. To toast pine nuts, place in a small skillet over medium-low heat and stir often for 3 to 4 minutes. Pine nuts are ready when they're an amber brown color.

PREPARE THE PESTO

Chop the garlic in a blender or food processor. Add pine nuts, basil, and salt and pulse until finely chopped. With the food processor running, add the oil, water or broth, and balsamic vinegar. Blend until nice and smooth and velvety green.

For the pesto:

1 garlic clove, crushed

⅓ cup pine nuts, toasted

2 cups loosely packed fresh basil leaves (usually one bunch of basil)

½ teaspoon salt

3 tablespoons olive oil

2 tablespoons water or vegetable broth

1 teaspoon balsamic vinegar

For the scramble:

2 tablespoons olive oil

1 small red onion, quartered and sliced (not too thin)

1 cup grape tomatoes

2 garlic cloves, minced

1 pound firm or extra-firm tofu

Fresh black pepper

PREPARE THE SCRAMBLE

Preheat a large skillet over medium-high heat. Add the oil and sauté the onion for about 3 minutes, until softened. Add the tomatoes and cook for about 5 minutes, stirring occasionally, until the tomatoes are cooked through and skins are starting to crinkle. Add the garlic and stir for about 30 seconds.

Squeeze the excess water out of the tofu and break it off into the pan in bite-size pieces. Take care not to make the pieces too small; they will break up a bit in the pan. Cook for about 10 minutes, tossing occasionally. Mix in the pesto and dashes of pepper. Cook until the pesto is heated through, about 2 minutes. Serve immediately.

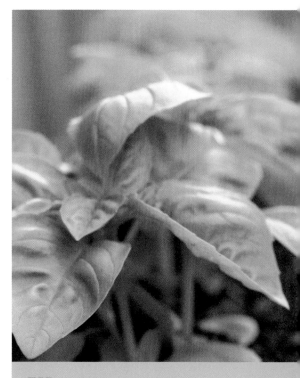

TIP When pulling the leaves from the basil, be careful to not get any stem into the pesto. Basil is one of those herbs where the stem can turn the whole thing bitter.

Cubed or Crumbled?

After moving to Portland, I came to know the cubed school of scrambled tofu. That is, the tofu is cut into squares and sautéed, instead of being crumbled up. Although I am a crumbled girl at heart, I can get down with the cubed variety. I'll admit that deciding if a scramble recipe was cubed or crumbled was part instinct but also rather arbitrary. Feel free to ignore me in these recipes and go with the tofu style you like best.

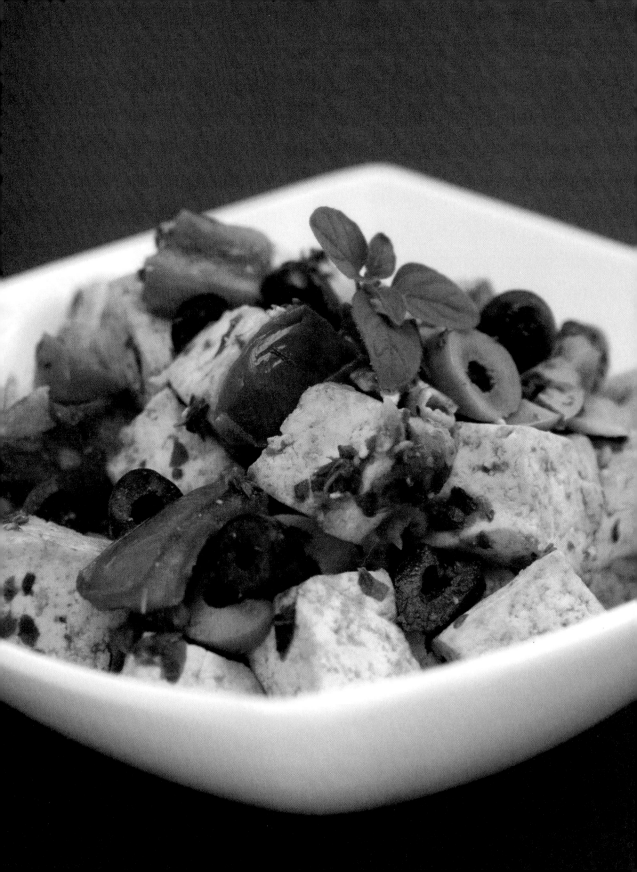

Puttanesca Scramble

Serves 4

Inspired by the classic Italian dish, pasta put-tanesca, this scramble is screaming with flavor. Olives, capers, and plenty of fresh herbs make for an easy-to-throw-together scramble that tastes like a Mediterranean feast you've been slaving over for hours. This pairs well with Potato Spinach Squares (page 116).

Preheat a large, heavy-bottomed pan over medium heat. Sauté the garlic in the olive oil until lightly browned, but be careful not to burn. Three minutes ought to do it. Add the red pepper flakes and the tofu and sauté for about 10 minutes, until tofu is browned. Add a little extra oil if necessary.

Mix in tomatoes, thyme, and oregano and cook for about 5 minutes, until tomatoes are a bit broken down but still whole. Add olives, capers, and salt. Cook just until heated through.

2 tablespoons olive oil

6–8 garlic cloves, thinly sliced

½ teaspoon crushed red pepper flakes

1 pound extra-firm tofu, diced

4 Roma tomatoes, diced

2 tablespoons fresh thyme

2 tablespoons fresh oregano

½ cup mixed olives, roughly chopped

1 tablespoon capers

¼ teaspoon salt, or to taste

Sesame Scrambled Tofu and Greens with Yams

Serves 4

Super simple but so yummy and satisfying, this is a throw-it-all-together kind of meal that incorporates all the great flavors: nutty, earthy, savory, spicy, and sweet. It calls for two baked yams, so put them in the oven at 350°F for about 40 minutes the night before, and let them cool in the fridge. It takes no time or effort at all! Well, minimum time and effort, anyway. For the greens, you can use any dark leafy greens, like kale, chard, or collards. I think red Swiss chard looks the prettiest and tastes pretty darn good, too.

1 tablespoon toasted sesame oil, plus extra for drizzling

4 garlic cloves, minced

1 tablespoon minced ginger

¼ teaspoon crushed red pepper flakes

1 pound extra-firm tofu

1 bunch leafy greens, chopped

2 tablespoons soy sauce

2 medium-size yams, baked, cooled, peeled, and cut into bite-size chunks

3 tablespoons toasted sesame seeds

Preheat a large pan over medium heat. Sauté garlic, ginger, and red pepper flakes in the oil for about a minute. Tear the tofu into bite-size pieces and add them to the pan. Turn the heat up and sauté for about 5 minutes, until the tofu is lightly browned.

Add the greens and soy sauce. Sauté for about 7 minutes, or until the greens have completely cooked down (collards may take longer than chard or kale). Splash some water into the pan if needed. Add the yams and gently stir just to cook through, being careful not to mush them too much.

Transfer scrambled tofu to bowls and drizzle each serving with additional sesame oil, maybe a teaspoon per serving. Sprinkle generously with sesame seeds and serve.

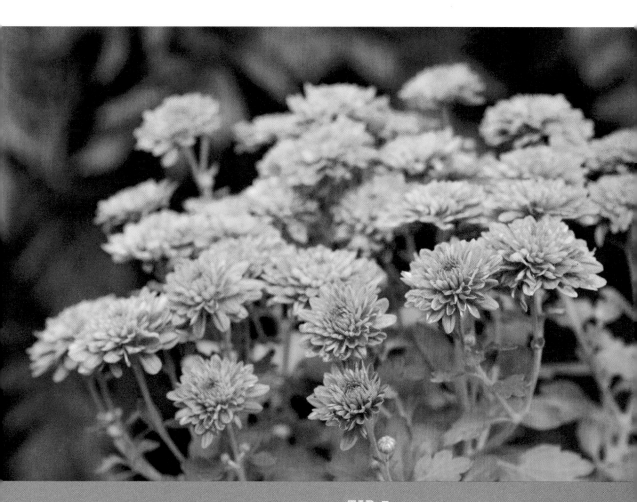

TIP To toast your own sesame seeds, preheat a small pan over medium heat. Gently heat the sesame seeds for about 3 minutes, stirring pretty constantly until they are toasty looking and aromatic. No need to get them all a uniform color; it's prettier when they are varying shades of brown. Remove from the heat as soon as they are done.

Scrambled Tortillas

Serves 4

It's a little difficult to describe this unique dish, but let me try: steamed tortillas are sautéed with onions and jalapeños and then coated in blended soft tofu. As everything cooks together, the tortillas are transformed into little morsels of heaven—the tofu firms around the outside and the tortilla remains tender on the inside. Then you toss in some steamed potatoes and ladle a tasty tomato sauce over the top. I like to stir the tomato sauce into the dish once it's already in my bowl and top with guacamole for good measure. It's the kind of comfort food that might not photograph well but is darn hard to stop eating. My recipe testers were skeptical at first, but they were won over once they tried it, and so shall you be.

Boil water for steaming. Steam the tortillas in a steaming basket for about 2 minutes, until soft and pliable. Remove from steam and set aside. Steam the potatoes for about 10 minutes, until tender but still firm.

Meanwhile, sauté the onion and jalapeños in oil in a large pan (preferably cast iron) over medium heat for 5 to 7 minutes. Add the tortillas, cumin, and salt and sauté for 5 more minutes.

Meanwhile, start the sauce in a saucepan. Sauté the garlic in oil until fragrant, about a minute. Add the cumin, oregano, chili powder, and salt and sauté for 30 seconds or so. Add tomato sauce and heat through. Add hot sauce if using, turn the heat off, and cover the sauce to keep it warm.

For the tortillas:

6 five-inch corn tortillas, torn into large strips (3 to 4 inches)

1 pound Yukon Gold potatoes, sliced about ¼ inch thick and 1 inch across

1 tablespoon olive oil

1 onion, thinly sliced

2 jalapeños, seeded and thinly sliced

½ teaspoon ground cumin

½ teaspoon salt

1 pound soft tofu, blended until smooth

For the sauce:

2 teaspoons olive oil

4 garlic cloves, minced

2 teaspoons ground cumin

1 tablespoon oregano

1 teaspoon chili powder

½ teaspoon salt

1 sixteen-ounce can tomato sauce

1 teaspoon hot sauce, or to taste (optional)

For serving:

Thinly chopped scallions for garnish (optional)

Guacamole (page 221, optional)

Back to the tortillas: pour the blended tofu over the tortillas and toss to coat. Raise the heat to medium high and sauté the tofu and tortillas for about 10 minutes more. Scrape the bottom of the pan to get the nice crusty bits and to make sure that you don't lose anything to the bottom of the pan. The dish is ready when the outsides of the tortillas are lightly browned and the tofu is firmer. Add the potatoes and toss to mix them in.

Scoop scrambled tortillas into a bowl and pour the sauce over the top. Sprinkle with scallions and top with guacamole if you like and serve.

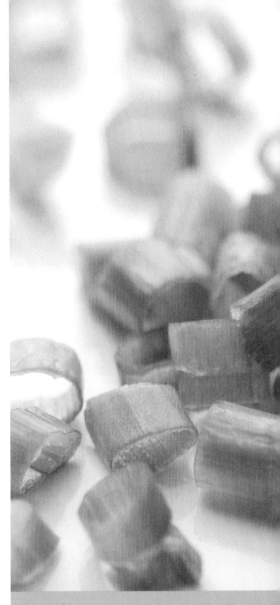

TIP Don't press the tofu before blending it; it needs moisture in order to get smooth. If it doesn't seem to be smoothing out add water by the tablespoon as you blend. And don't forget, use soft tofu! Not extra-firm or silken.

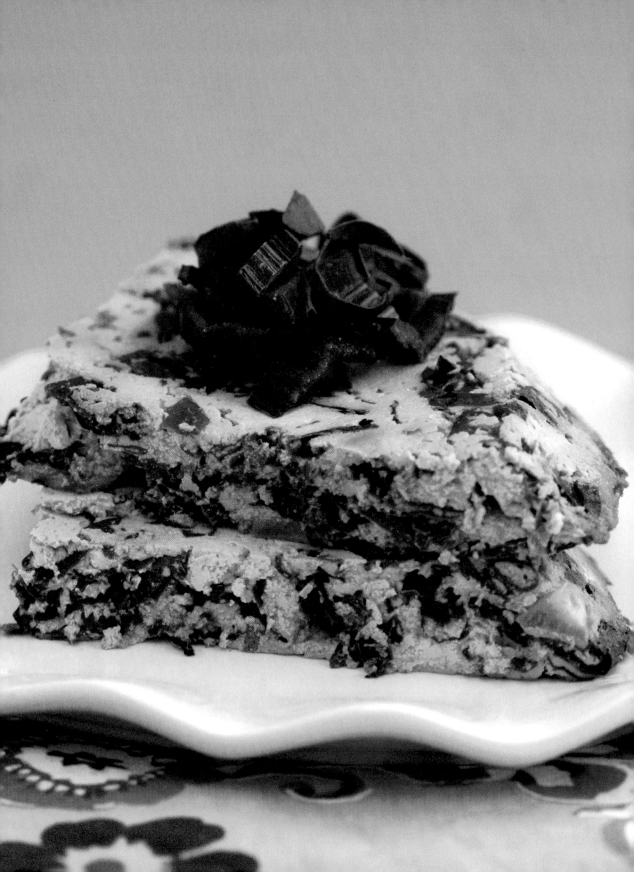

Swiss Chard Frittata

Serves 4

The deep, earthy taste of Swiss chard is intensified and made sweeter with thinly sliced garlic, rather than minced. Use red Swiss chard if you can find it because it leaves pretty fuchsia flecks in the frittata.

1 tablespoon olive oil

6 garlic cloves, thinly sliced

1 bunch red Swiss chard, rough stems removed, chopped well (about 4 cups)

2 teaspoons dried oregano

1 pound firm or extra-firm tofu

1 tablespoon soy sauce

1 teaspoon prepared mustard (Dijon or yellow, whatever you got)

¼ teaspoon turmeric

Several dashes fresh black pepper

¼ cup nutritional yeast

Salt, to taste

Preheat the oven to 400°F.

Preheat a large, heavy-bottomed pan over medium-low heat. Add the oil and the garlic and cook for about 3 minutes, stirring occasionally. What you're doing here is "blonding" the garlic—it's ready when it's turned a light amber color.

Add the chard and oregano and turn up the heat to medium high. Sauté the chard for about 5 minutes, until it is completely wilted. Add splashes of water if needed to get the chard to cook down.

Meanwhile, while the chard is cooking, prepare your frittata base. Give the tofu a squeeze over the sink to remove some of the water. Use your hands to crumble and squeeze it in a large mixing bowl, until it has the consistency of ricotta cheese (about 3 minutes). Add the soy sauce, mustard, turmeric, black pepper, and yeast to the tofu and mix well. When your chard is ready, incorporate it into the tofu. Be sure to get all of the garlic, but if there is any water in the pan try to avoid adding it to the tofu. Taste for salt.

Lightly grease an 8-inch pie plate and firmly press your frittata mixture into it. Bake for 20 minutes, until

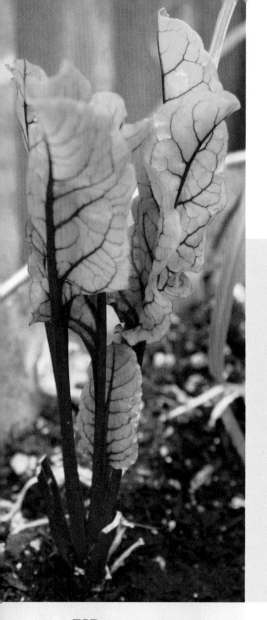

the frittata is firm and lightly browned on top. Let cool for about 3 minutes, then invert onto a plate and serve.

Feel Free to Frittata

A frittata is an open-faced omelet. In our case, it's akin to a casserole that is perfect for slicing and serving with potatoes and a salad. What I love about it is not only that it's the perfect vehicle for delivering scrumptious ingredients, like shiitakes or greens, but that because a lot of the cooking time is spent in the oven, it frees up your stove top for other things like dancing on it or, I don't know, making home fries and pancakes. Frittatas also reheat beautifully or taste great at room temperature. It's as if they are just daring you to come up with a reason not to make one.

TIP Use the stems of the chard, but discard the very lower part where they are a little too woody to cook properly. Just make sure to thinly slice the upper part of the stem that you do use. You can also save some of the thinly sliced stems to use as garnish.

Shiitake Dill Frittata

Serves 4

The mushroom-dill combination is one of my favorites. I commonly use cremini or button mushrooms, but I used shiitake in this recipe to switch things up and add a chewy bite to the frittata.

Preheat the oven to 400°F.

Preheat a large, heavy-bottomed pan over medium-low heat. Sauté the garlic in olive oil until fragrant, about 30 seconds. Add the shiitake mushrooms and cook until softened, stirring occasionally, about 7 minutes.

Meanwhile, prepare your frittata base. Give the tofu a squeeze over the sink to remove a little of the water. Use your hands to crumble and squeeze it in a large mixing bowl, until it has the consistency of ricotta cheese (about 3 minutes). Make sure to mash it really well, leaving no large chunks, or you may have issues with getting it out of the pan in one piece. Add the soy sauce, mustard, turmeric, black pepper, yeast, and dill to the tofu and mix well. When the mushrooms are ready, incorporate the mushroom mixture into the tofu. Taste for salt.

Lightly grease an 8-inch pie plate and firmly press your frittata mixture into it. Bake for 20 minutes, until the frittata is firm and lightly browned on top. Let cool for about 3 minutes, then invert onto a plate and serve.

1 tablespoon olive oil

4 garlic cloves, minced

6 ounces shiitake mushrooms, thinly sliced (2 cups)

1 pound firm or extra-firm tofu

1 tablespoon soy sauce

1 teaspoon prepared mustard (Dijon or yellow, whatever you got)

¼ teaspoon turmeric

Several dashes fresh black pepper

¼ cup nutritional yeast

½ cup loosely packed chopped fresh dill

¼ teaspoon salt, or to taste

Curried Cauliflower Frittata

Serves 4

Cauliflower and curry just love each other. It's very important that you cut the cauliflower very small so that the frittata holds together, so thinly slice the stems and make sure that the florets are no more than ½ inch long. Depending on the spiciness of your curry powder, you might want to start with a little less than 2 tablespoons and work your way up.

Preheat the oven to 400°F.

Preheat a large, heavy-bottomed pan over medium-high heat. Sauté the cauliflower in oil for about 10 minutes, until softened and lightly browned. Add splashes of water if it starts to appear dry. Add the garlic and sauté another minute.

Now prepare your frittata base. Give the tofu a squeeze over the sink to remove some of the water. Use your hands to crumble and squeeze it in a large mixing bowl, until it has the consistency of ricotta cheese (about 3 minutes). Add the remaining ingredients to the tofu and mix well. You can grate the carrot directly into the mixture with a box grater. When your cauliflower is ready, incorporate it into the tofu. Be sure to get all of the garlic. Taste for salt, lemon, and seasoning.

1 tablespoon peanut oil

2 cups finely chopped cauliflower

4 garlic cloves, minced

1 pound firm or extra-firm tofu

1 tablespoon soy sauce

1 tablespoon fresh lemon juice,
    from about half a lemon

2 tablespoons curry powder

½ teaspoon ground cumin

¼ cup nutritional yeast

1 small carrot, peeled and grated

¼ teaspoon salt, or to taste

Lemon to taste

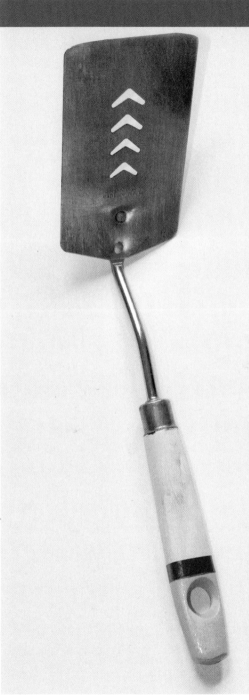

Lightly grease an 8-inch pie plate and firmly press your frittata mixture into it. Bake for 20 minutes, until the frittata is firm and lightly browned on top. Let cool for about 3 minutes, then invert onto a plate and serve.

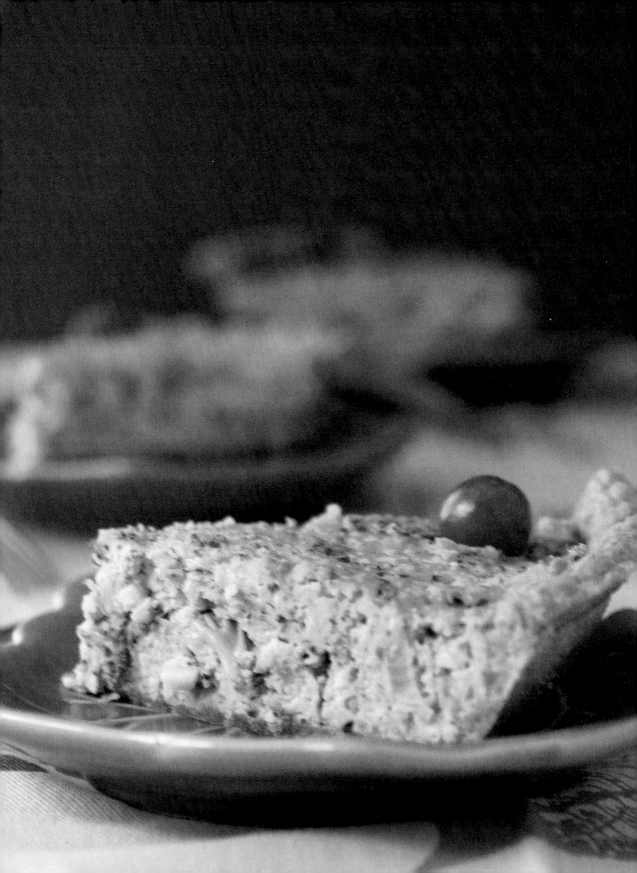

Classic Broccoli Quiche

Serves 6 to 8

Everything about quiche is appealing, from its spelling (it's got a Q!) to its shape (it's a pie!) to its color (who doesn't love the '70s?). I also like that it's delicious served at room temperature and reheats wonderfully. In this recipe, cashews help us to achieve the creaminess that people expect from quiche. Serve with a crisp green salad and maybe some Sausages (pages 137–140) if you're in the mood.

Make ahead: You can make the quiche up to two days before serving it. After cooking, let cool a bit, then wrap tightly in plastic wrap. To reheat, place in a preheated 350°F oven for 15 to 20 minutes.

Preheat the oven to 350°F. If using a homemade crust, roll the dough out into a 9-inch pie plate. Poke the bottom of the dough with a fork about five times to prevent it from puffing up, then bake for 10 minutes and remove from oven. In the meantime, start preparing the filling.

Preheat a large, heavy-bottomed skillet (preferably cast iron) over medium heat. Sauté the onion and garlic in the oil for about 3 minutes. Add the broccoli, thyme, tarragon, turmeric, salt, and pepper. Cook for 10 minutes, until broccoli is soft. If it starts to look dry add a tablespoon or two of water.

Meanwhile, in a food processor, pulse the cashews into fine crumbs. Give the tofu a squeeze to remove some of the water, then crumble it into the food pro-

2 tablespoons olive oil

1 medium onion, finely chopped

3 garlic cloves, minced

3 cups finely chopped broccoli (see note)

1 teaspoon dried thyme

½ teaspoon dried tarragon

½ teaspoon turmeric

1 teaspoon salt

A healthy dose of fresh-cracked black pepper

½ cup raw, unsalted cashews

1 pound extra-firm tofu

1 teaspoon prepared mustard (Dijon or regular, most anything will work)

A handful of cherry or grape tomatoes for decorating (optional)

1 nine-inch pie crust, store-bought or homemade (see Basic Pastry Crust, page 47)

cessor along with the mustard. Process until relatively smooth. When the broccoli mixture is done cooking, add one cup of it to the food processor and pulse a few times to combine.

Transfer cashew mixture to a mixing bowl, add the rest of the broccoli mixture, and combine. Taste for salt. Use a rubber spatula to get everything into the pie crust and to smooth the top out. Place cherry tomatoes around the perimeter of the pie and one in the center for maximum *Good Housekeeping* adorableness. Bake for 40 minutes, until edges of the pie are lightly browned.

I suggest letting the quiche sit for 20 minutes before you dig in. I think it tastes best when it is moderately warm, not piping hot. It's also great at room temperature.

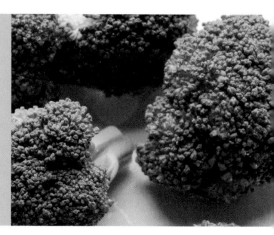

TIP The broccoli pieces should be tiny, anywhere between the size of a pea to the size of a dime. As you chop, the florets might become crumbs. That's just fine! Scrape them up with your knife and use them.

I love using baby tomatoes of any sort to decorate the quiche. While they do taste great baked, my main objective is to bring a little color to the dish. You can also use thinly sliced tomatoes, red bell pepper rings, or roasted red peppers.

❀ VARIATION ❀

CAULIFLOWER AND RED BELL PEPPER QUICHE

Replace broccoli with **cauliflower**. Add **1 finely chopped red bell pepper** when you sauté the onion.

Caramelized Vidalia Onion Quiche

Serves 6 to 8

Sometimes the simplest ingredients make the best-tasting food. With this rich quiche, it's all about the method. Caramelizing the onions gives them such lip-smacking depth that adding anything else would just take away from the flavor. Serve with a salad for a simple and classy meal.

Preheat the oven to 350°F. If using a homemade crust, roll the dough out into a 9-inch pie plate. Poke the bottom of the dough with a fork about five times to prevent it from puffing up, then bake for 10 minutes and remove from oven. In the meantime, start preparing the filling.

Preheat a heavy-bottomed skillet, preferably cast iron, over low heat. Add the oil and the onions and toss the onions to coat. Cover and cook for 20 minutes, leaving a little gap for steam to escape. Stir occasionally, every 5 minutes or so. Onions should turn a nice, mellow amber color, but not burn, although a couple of darker spots are fine.

Remove the lid and turn up the heat just a bit, to a medium setting. Stir often for 10 more minutes. Onions should become darker in color, and some of the moisture should evaporate.

Meanwhile, process the cashews in a food processor into fine crumbs. Add the salt and nutmeg. Give

2 tablespoons olive oil

3 to 4 Vidalia onions, diced medium (about 3 pounds; you can also use Walla Walla or another sweet onion)

¾ cup raw, unsalted cashews

1 teaspoon salt

¼ teaspoon ground nutmeg

1 pound extra-firm tofu

1 nine-inch pie crust, store-bought or homemade (see Basic Pastry Crust, page 47)

the tofu a squeeze to get rid of some of the water, then crumble it into the food processor. Process until relatively smooth. If it seems to be too thick and not pureeing, add a tablespoon of water or two. When the caramelized onions are done cooking, add a ½ cup of them to the food processor and pulse a few times to combine.

Transfer cashew mixture to a mixing bowl and mix in the rest of the onions. Taste for salt. Use a rubber spatula to get everything into the pie crust and smooth the top out. Bake for 40 minutes, until edges of the pie are lightly browned.

I suggest letting the quiche sit for 20 minutes before you dig in. I think it tastes best when it is moderately warm, rather than piping hot. It's also great at room temperature.

Caramelized Onions

This is kind of an art, so don't rush it! Since the onions can be left alone for intervals, you can prep the rest of your recipe while the onions caramelize. The basic idea here is to sweat the onions, which means you'll be gently cooking them covered over low heat, and a lot of the cooking will be done from the steam as the water is released. You're coaxing the sweetness out of them and locking it in. It looks like a lot of onion, and it is, but everything will cook down to manageable proportions. If you've never tasted caramelized onions, you might be surprised that an onion is even capable of this deep flavor.

Mushroom, Leek, and White Bean Pie

Serves 6 to 8

This pie was inspired by my need for a tofuless quiche. It has a comforting Thanksgiving taste that is perfect for autumn mornings. Serve with Roasted Root Vegetables (page 145) to seal the deal.

Preheat the oven to 350°F. Thinly slice 4 mushrooms and set them aside. They'll be used to decorate the top of the pie. Roughly chop the remainder of the mushrooms.

Preheat a large, heavy-bottomed skillet over medium heat. Sauté the leeks in the olive oil for about 3 minutes. Add the mushrooms and sauté for about 7 minutes more, until the moisture has released and they're nice and soft. Add the garlic, thyme, and pepper; sauté for another minute; then remove from heat.

Your oven should be preheated by now, so poke the bottom of the pie crust with a fork about five times to prevent it from puffing up, then bake for 10 minutes and remove from oven.

Now, prepare the filling. Pulse the walnuts in a food processor until fine crumbs form. Add the beans and a tablespoon of water and blend. If the beans aren't blending easily, add another tablespoon of water. Add the cornstarch and salt. Blend until the cornstarch isn't visible.

1 pound cremini mushrooms

2 tablespoons olive oil

3 cups thickly sliced leeks (white and green parts)

3 garlic cloves, chopped

Heaping tablespoon chopped fresh thyme

Fresh black pepper

1 cup shelled walnuts

1 fifteen-ounce can cannellini beans (1½ cups cooked), drained and rinsed

1 to 2 tablespoons water

2 tablespoons cornstarch

¾ teaspoon salt

A few sprigs of thyme for decoration

1 nine-inch pie crust, store-bought or homemade (see Basic Pastry Crust, page 47)

Add the leek mixture to the food processor. Use a spoon to mix it into the beans before you start processing. You're going to be pulsing the mixture up but not completely blending it in, so it's important to incorporate it beforehand. Now pulse a few times, so that the leeks and mushrooms are still visible, but chopped into small bits.

Spoon the filling into the prebaked crust, smoothing the top with the back of a spoon. Press the reserved mushroom slices into the perimeter of the quiche and press a few sprigs of thyme down the center.

Bake for 40 minutes. Let cool for at least 30 minutes before serving. This quiche tastes great at room temperature.

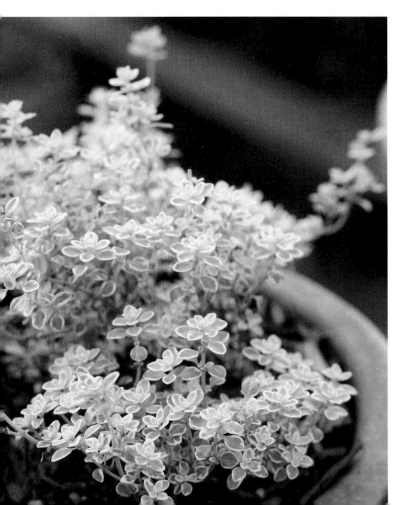

Basic Pastry Crust

A tender and flaky crust, perfect for quiche. The crust is very versatile; use it not just for quiches (pages 41–44) or the Mushroom, Leek, and White Bean Pie (page 45), but next time you're making an apple pie.

1½ cups all-purpose flour

Large pinch sea salt

¼ cup chilled margarine

5 to 6 tablespoons chilled water

Sift the flour and the salt into a large mixing bowl. Add the margarine in small chunks to the flour. Use a pastry knife to cut it into the flour until it resembles coarse crumbs. Add the water in tablespoonfuls until the pastry begins to hold together. Gather it into a ball. Wrap with plastic wrap and place in the fridge for about 45 minutes.

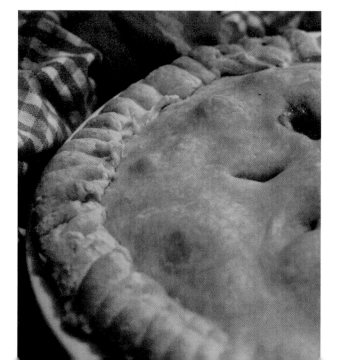

Fennel Breakfast Risotto

Serves 6

I have a long-standing love affair with rice for breakfast, but I could never get behind those quaint recipes that tell you to eat sweetened rice and cinnamon like you would oatmeal. No thanks, save the rice pudding for dessert. Savory is where it's at. Risotto may seem like a bit too much stirring for the morning, but have your coffee, put on some music, and go for it—I promise it's worth the effort. Spiked with fennel for a bit of a sausage-y flavor, this melt-in-your-mouth risotto is a warm auburn color. It's delicious as an entree, served in bowls and topped with Smoky Shiitakes (page 150), or as a side dish instead of potatoes.

6 cups vegetable broth

1 tablespoon olive oil

1 large red bell pepper, seeds removed, finely chopped

1½ cups finely chopped shallots

4 garlic cloves, minced

2 tablespoons fennel seeds, chopped

1 teaspoon dried thyme

A few dashes fresh black pepper

1 cup dry white wine

½ teaspoon salt

1½ cups Arborio rice

4 leaves fresh sage, chopped (optional)

Warm the vegetable broth in a saucepan. Keep it warm on the lowest setting possible as you prepare the risotto.

Preheat a heavy-bottomed soup pot over medium heat. Sauté the red bell pepper and shallots in the oil for about 10 minutes. Add the garlic, fennel seeds, thyme, and pepper and sauté 2 minutes more.

Add the wine and salt, then turn the heat up so that the wine boils and reduces—about 2 minutes. Lower the heat back to medium.

Add the rice and stir for about 2 minutes. The rice should soak up the liquid from the pot and become light brown. Add the broth by the cupful, stirring the risotto after each addition until the broth is mostly absorbed (6 to 8 minutes). If the broth isn't absorbing, raise the heat a bit. It absorbs faster as the rice gets more and more tender.

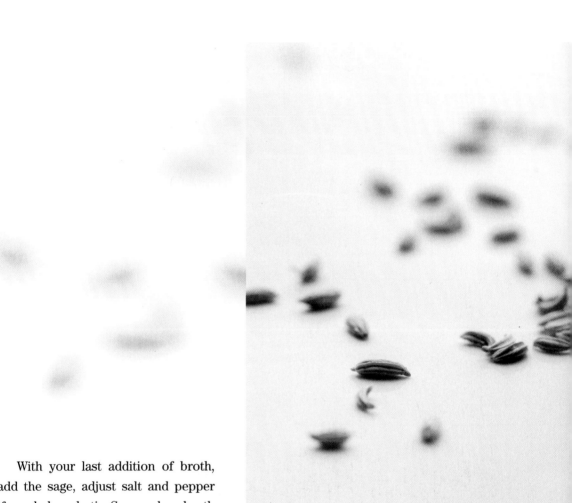

With your last addition of broth, add the sage, adjust salt and pepper if needed, and stir. Serve when broth is mostly absorbed but the rice is still creamy.

TIP If you have leftover risotto, or just want an interesting side dish, form cooled risotto into patties and lightly fry in olive oil on both sides until heated through.

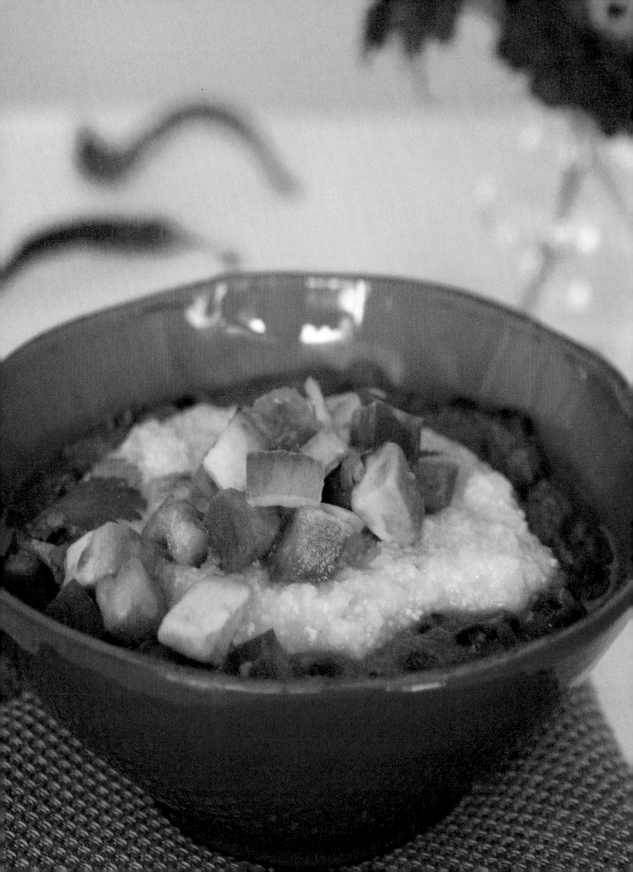

Polenta Rancheros

Serves 4 to 6

This might have been my first-ever brunch invention way back when I was a teenager. I really missed the softness of an egg over saucy rancheros beans. Creamy polenta really does the trick, plus has the added benefit of delicate corn flavor that fits in just right. This recipe is really simple but can be fancied up by adding Cashew Sour Cream (page 211) and a big spoonful of Guacamole (page 221). A cherry tomato on top couldn't hurt, either. The Creamy Avocado Potato Salad (page 123) makes a great accompaniment, too. If you time everything right the recipe should take about half an hour; just start toasting the seeds for the sauce while you boil the broth for the polenta.

PREPARE THE BEANS AND SAUCE

Preheat a large, heavy-bottomed pan, preferably cast iron, over medium heat. Dry toast the seeds in the pan for about 2 minutes, stirring frequently, until they're fragrant and a few shades darker (just be careful not to burn them). Raise the heat to medium high, add the oil, and sauté the onion, peppers, and garlic for about 10 minutes, until onion is browned. Add the tomato sauce, salt, and syrup and cook for about 5 minutes.

Transfer the onion mixture to a blender or food processor and blend until smooth. If using a blender, intermittently lift the lid to let steam escape so that it doesn't build up and explode.

For the rancheros sauce and beans:

2 teaspoons cumin seeds

2 teaspoons coriander seeds

2 tablespoons oil

1 large yellow onion, diced medium

2 Serrano peppers, seeded and chopped

4 garlic cloves, chopped

1 fifteen-ounce can tomato sauce

½ teaspoon salt

1 teaspoon pure maple syrup or agave nectar

2 fifteen-ounce cans black beans, drained and rinsed

For the soft polenta:

5 cups vegetable broth

½ teaspoon salt

1 cup polenta cornmeal

2 tablespoons olive oil

Optional items for garnish:

Chopped green onions

Cashew Sour Cream (page 211)

Guacamole (page 221)

Cherry tomatoes

Buying polenta in this day and age might send you into a tailspin. Different packages may say different things but contain the same product. Sometimes the label says "polenta cornmeal," sometimes it says "polenta corn grits," sometimes it just says "cornmeal," sometimes it just says "polenta," and sometimes it doesn't say polenta at all but "Alien Fairy Dust," yet it does indeed contain polenta. Why do they do this? My best guess is they want to make Italian cooking only accessible to grandmas throughout Brooklyn. But the fact of the matter is that polenta is cornmeal. The only suggestion I would make is not to buy the finely ground variety. Instead, stick to the coarse-ground or to packages that do clearly state that it's polenta inside. I find that finely ground cornmeal won't give the fluffy results we're looking for. My favorite brand, and one that is widely available, is Bob's Red Mill, whose label states "Corn Grits, also known as Polenta," in case there is any doubt.

Return the sauce to the pan and add the beans. Cook over medium heat until the beans are heated through, about 5 minutes.

PREPARE THE POLENTA

In a saucepan, bring the broth and salt to a boil. Add the polenta in a slow, steady stream, whisking as you pour it. Add the olive oil and lower the heat to simmer. Let cook for 12 minutes, stirring often. Turn off the heat, cover, and let sit for 10 more minutes, stirring occasionally.

TO SERVE

I like to use wide, shallow bowls for this dish, but any bowl should be just fine. Ladle some beans into the bowl and top with a big spoonful of polenta. Dot with the sour cream by drizzling drops slowly from a tablespoon, and top with a dollop of guacamole. Finish it off with chopped green onions and a cherry tomato. Voilà!

TIP You'll have more polenta than you need for this recipe, but put the extra in an airtight container and refrigerate. The next morning, lightly fry it on both sides for a breakfast treat.

Matzoh Brie

Serves 4

If you're Jewish or a New Yorker at all, you'll be really happy to have a workable vegan matzoh brie recipe. Maybe your mouth is already watering at the thought of the softened matzoh, lightly fried and spiked with just a few fried onions. If you aren't Jewish or a New Yorker, I am going to be honest and say that sometimes I have a really hard time explaining Jewish food in a way that makes it sound appealing to non-Jews. Often I read things on the Internet that say some of my recipes are "weird" and "ethnic." I'll just invite you skeptics to loosen up and try this— it is classic Jewish comfort food! Diner Home Fries (page 117) or Red Flannel Hash (page 119) and a salad make the meal complete.

6 matzohs, lightly salted and preferably whole wheat

2 tablespoons olive oil

1 medium onion, thinly sliced

½ pound soft tofu, blended until smooth

¾ teaspoon salt

½ teaspoon ground black pepper

A handful chopped fresh dill for garnish

Break the matzoh into pieces that are about 1½ to 2 inches big. Place them in a bowl and cover with warm tap water. Let them soak for 3 to 5 minutes, until they are softened but not falling apart. (Check them after 3 minutes; they should be flexible but still intact.) Then drain the matzoh in a colander.

In the meantime, preheat a large skillet over medium-high heat. Sauté the onion in the oil for about 7 minutes, until the onion is browned and slightly caramelized. Add the matzoh and tofu and use a spatula to coat the matzoh with the tofu. Add salt and pepper. Cook the mixture for about 10 minutes, flipping often, until the matzoh is browned and most of the tofu has been cooked dry. I usually let it brown for a few minutes, use a spatula to cut it into pieces, then flip those pieces.

Serve topped with chopped fresh dill.

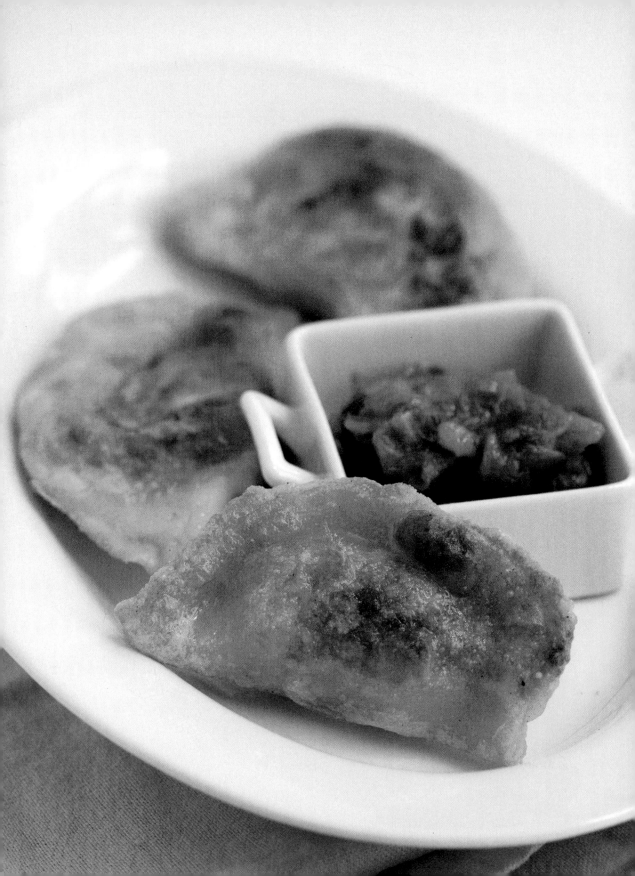

Pierogi (Potato and Mushroom Sauerkraut)

Makes around 30 pierogi

Everyone's favorite Polish dumpling. Toothsome, warm, soft, and smothered in caramelized onions—yep, that's the stuff! In NYC, pierogi are a brunch staple. Our Polish diners are a disappearing breed, but you can live the life in your own kitchen.

This is one of those time-consuming recipes that will change your life. If you make them once and know what to expect, the next time you make them won't be such a big deal. Because the ingredients are so simple and unadulterated, choose good-quality, organic potatoes whose flavor packs the most punch.

MAKE THE
CARAMELIZED ONIONS

Preheat a heavy-bottomed skillet, preferably cast iron, over low heat. Add the oil and the onions and toss the onions to coat. Cover and cook for 20 minutes, leaving a little gap for steam to escape. Stir occasionally, every 5 minutes or so. Onions should turn amber, but not burn, although a couple of darker spots are fine (see box, page 44).

For the caramelized onions:

¼ cup canola oil

2 pounds sweet onions (Vidalia or Walla Walla), diced medium

For the potato filling:

1½ pounds Yukon Gold potatoes, peeled and sliced, cut into ¾-inch chunks

¼ cup canola oil

1 small onion, finely chopped

½ teaspoon salt

½ teaspoon pepper

For the mushroom sauerkraut filling:

4 tablespoons nonhydrogenated margarine (or ¼ cup canola oil and ¼ teaspoon salt)

10 ounces mushrooms, sliced (about 3 cups)

2 cups sauerkraut

¼ teaspoon pepper

For the dough:

1 cup warm water

3 tablespoons canola oil

3 cups all-purpose flour, divided, plus a little extra for sprinkling

¾ teaspoon salt

For serving:

Applesauce

Remove the cover and turn the heat up just a bit, to a medium setting. Stir often for 10 more minutes. Onions should become a darker amber, and some of the moisture should evaporate.

MAKE THE POTATO FILLING

In a medium-size pot, cover potatoes in water. Place a lid on the pot and bring to a boil. Once boiling, cook for about 20 more minutes or until potatoes are easily pierced with a fork.

Meanwhile, in a large pan, sauté the onions in oil over medium heat for about 7 minutes. Turn the heat off but continue to stir occasionally because they could still burn from the hot pan. When the potatoes are done boiling, drain them well and add them to the pan with the onions. Just mash them right in there with a potato masher; that way you are sure to get all the oil, plus you save a dish. Add the salt and pepper. Make sure potatoes are mashed well and fluffy. Set aside to cool a bit.

MAKE THE MUSHROOM SAUERKRAUT FILLING

You know I don't usually advise cooking with margarine, but I really love it with the mushrooms here, I think because growing up the mushrooms I ate were really buttery. Anyway, this filling is really simple. In a large skillet, melt the margarine over medium-high heat. Add the mushrooms and sauté for about 7 minutes, until the mushrooms are soft.

Before adding the sauerkraut to the pan, give it a squeeze over the sink to get out as much water as you can. It's important to do this so that your pierogi don't get all wet. You'll need to add the sauerkraut to the pan a cup at a time. Add to the pan and cook for about 10 minutes, cooking out any excess water. Season with the pepper. The filling shouldn't look dry (a small amount of water is okay), but you shouldn't be able to slosh around in it in rain boots.

MAKE THE DOUGH

This is really the brunt of the work in this recipe. If you're like me, you have limited counter space and so rolling out dough can be a hassle. I make the dough last because the mess becomes much more manageable when you don't have to prep on the counter afterwards. It also gives your filling some time to cool. So make sure you clean up after your filling making and get someone to do the dishes for you. I find that a serene counter makes all the difference in dough making.

Pour the water and oil into a large bowl. Add 2 cups of the flour and the salt, keeping one cup aside. Use a fork to stir the flour in, and as it starts to come together, use your hands to knead until a loose dough forms (about 3 minutes).

Sprinkle your counter with flour, then turn the dough out onto it and knead. Add the reserved cup of flour a little bit at a time, working it into the dough, until it is very smooth and elastic, about 10 minutes. If it's too sticky, you can add a little bit more flour and knead it in, sometimes up to ¼ cup extra. Conversely, if you get a good-feeling, smooth, elastic dough with less than the extra cup of flour, then that's okay, too.

Now we roll the dough out, and also bring a salted pot of water to boil—the largest pot you've got—for boiling the pierogi.

Divide the dough in half and make sure your counter is clean and sprinkled with a dusting of flour to prevent sticking. Roll half the dough out to about $\frac{1}{16}$ of an inch thick, which is to say, very thin but not see-through. I roll it into an 18×10-inch rectangle, but as long as you have the thinness going, the shape doesn't matter so much. Sprinkle the top with a light dusting of flour.

Now we're going to make circles. I use the top of a glass that is 3½ inches in diameter, but somewhere between 3½ and 4 inches is perfect. Use a glass or a cookie cutter. Have ready a lightly floured plate to place the finished circles on, and go ahead and firmly press your glass or cookie cutter into the dough, as close together as you can. Pull together the excess dough and set aside. Place circles on the floured plate and transfer to the fridge while you repeat with the other half of the dough. Combine the excess dough and see if you can get a few more wrappers out of the deal.

Note: If it's very hot in your kitchen there's a chance that the circles will stick together. Sprinkle them with flour and make sure they don't get wet to prevent sticking. If they do stick, you can roll them out and try again.

BOIL THE PIEROGI

Now we're ready to boil some pierogi! Make sure your water is rapidly boiling. The filling should be room temp or colder. Have a small bowl of water for wetting the edges of the wrappers. Place about a tablespoon of filling into the center of a circle and dab water around the circumference of the circle. Fold the edges of the wrapper over filling and pinch in the middle to hold together. Pinch down the sides so that you have a sealed half-moon. Don't be shy with the pinching and don't try to make it look like perfect pinches. The most important thing is that you are getting them sealed, so use pressure and really seal them up. I think it looks really cool when the pinches aren't perfectly spaced; it gives them a beautiful homemade, rustic look and lets you know that it came from a person, not a robot.

If some of the filling is sneaking its way out, then use a little less filling with the next one. Once you get the amount of dough down, you can do a few at a time in conveyer belt style. I usually do six, lay out the circles, add the filling, pinch them closed. This works out perfectly if you time it with the boiling.

To boil, gently lower the pierogi into the water with a slotted spoon. Boil about six at a time. When they float they are ready. If for some reason they aren't floating, it takes about 4 minutes for them to cook. Use a slotted spoon to transfer them to a plate as you prepare the rest. Cover finished ones lightly with tin foil to keep warm. Proceed until all pierogi are boiled.

Now, I'm going to say something a lot of people might not want to hear or that you will at least severely disagree with. I don't think you should fry the pierogi. I think it's wrong in every way. But if you must, you can preheat a heavy-bottomed skillet over medium-high heat, add a thin layer of canola oil, and fry the pierogi on each side until golden brown (probably 3 minutes on one side and 1 minute on the other).

Serve the pierogi in an oversized bowl, sprinkled amply with salt and smothered in lots and lots of caramelized onions.

Beer-Battered Tofu

Serves 4 to 6

If totally *fried* and *greasy* and *yum* is what you crave in the morning, then this is the recipe for you. It's a thick, fish-'n'-chips-type batter, so since you're frying, might as well make some French fries to go along with it. Serve with malt vinegar and please the Britophile in you.

1 pound extra-firm tofu, drained and pressed

2 tablespoons soy sauce

Vegetable oil for frying

1 cup all-purpose flour

1 tablespoon cornstarch

¼ teaspoon baking powder

½ cup cold dark beer

½ cup cold water

Salt for sprinkling

Lay out some paper towels or brown paper bags for absorbing the oil.

Slice the tofu into eight pieces widthwise, then slice those pieces corner to corner, so that you have long triangles. Splash the soy sauce onto a plate and dredge the tofu slices in it. You can sprinkle on a little more if needed. Set the plate aside to let the tofu absorb the soy sauce while you prepare the batter.

Now you're going to preheat the oil, but first, assemble all your batter ingredients so that you can get that together while the oil is heating. Preheat a large, heavy-bottomed pan (preferably cast iron) over medium heat. Pour in about a half inch of oil. Proceed to make the batter.

In a large mixing bowl, use a fork to combine the flour, cornstarch, and baking powder. Make a well in the center of the flour and pour in the beer and water. Mix together until thoroughly combined. Test the oil by dropping in a drop of the batter; if rapid bubbles form around it then the oil is hot enough. If you have a thermometer then it should read between 325°F and 350°F.

Fry the tofu in two batches by thoroughly coating the tofu slices in batter and slipping them carefully into the hot oil. Fry tofu for about 3 minutes on one side and 2 on the other, or until golden. Place on paper towels to drain. Sprinkle with salt while still hot. If you need to keep the tofu slices warm for up to an hour, place in a 200°F oven until ready to serve.

Cornbread Waffles with Pantry Mole Rojo and Seitan

Serves 6

A fluffy-on-the-inside, crispy-on-the-outside cornmeal waffle is topped with sautéed seitan, bell peppers, and onions and smothered in a rich mole. There is no better way to introduce you to the world of savory waffles. Traditional mole rojo calls for a bunch of peppers that you might not have lying around, so this is a bastardized but delicious version using ingredients that are more common to, if not everyone's pantry, at least mine. The laundry list of ingredients looks daunting, but don't be afraid; it's mostly spices and the actual preparation is super simple.

Make ahead: Prepare the waffles the night before and refrigerate. Toast when ready to serve. The mole can be prepared the night before and gently reheated the day of.

For the mole rojo:

2 tablespoons olive oil

1 onion, diced medium

3 garlic cloves, minced

5 teaspoons chili powder

2 teaspoons dried oregano or marjoram

1 teaspoon ground cinnamon

¼ teaspoon ground allspice

1 teaspoon smoked paprika

1 fourteen-ounce can diced tomatoes

2 cups vegetable broth

3 tablespoons natural peanut butter

¼ cup raisins

½ cup crushed tortilla chips

½ cup slivered almonds

⅓ cup semi-sweet chocolate chips

For the sautéed seitan:

2 tablespoons olive oil

8 ounces seitan, thinly sliced
(about 2 cups)

1 red onion, sliced into half-
moons

1 yellow bell pepper, cut into
long strips

To serve:

1 recipe Cornbread Waffles,
savory variation (page 92)

Sliced avocado or Guacamole
(page 221)

Cilantro or finely chopped
scallions

TO MAKE THE MOLE

Preheat a soup pot over medium heat. Sauté the onions
in oil for 5 to 7 minutes, until onions are translucent. Add
the garlic, herbs, and spices. Sauté for another minute
or so.

Add the tomatoes and broth and bring to a boil. Once
boiling, add the peanut butter, raisins, and tortilla chips.
Simmer for about 15 minutes, until slightly reduced. In
the meantime, grind almonds in a food processor or
blender.

Once the mole has cooked for 15 minutes, transfer it
to a food processor or blender and puree until smooth. If
your blender isn't equipped with a lid that has an opening
on top, make sure to lift the lid every few seconds so that
the steam doesn't build up and explode.

Transfer the mole back to the pot and stir in the chocolate chips until they melt. Let sit for at least 10 minutes
so that the flavors marry. Taste and adjust seasoning if
necessary.

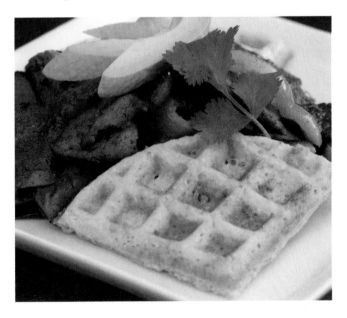

TO MAKE THE SEITAN

Preheat a large pan (preferably cast iron) over medium-high heat. Sauté everything in the oil until the seitan is slightly browned and the peppers are a little charred, about 15 minutes.

TO ASSEMBLE

If using round waffles, quarter and place overlapping, all pointing in the same direction. Top with seitan and then pour mole over everything. Top with avocado and garnishes.

❈ VARIATION ❈

Skip the sautéed seitan and friends and use two 15-ounce cans of rinsed and drained pinto beans (about 3 cups) instead.

TIP To get the timing right, make the mole first. While it's cooking, make the seitan. In your downtime, get together the ingredients for the waffles. I don't actually cook the waffles until everything else is done, just for the sake of sanity, but you can definitely measure out all of the waffle ingredients beforehand.

For even more flavor, toast the slivered almonds in a pan over medium heat until they turn a few shades darker. Not totally necessary if you're feeling lazy, but a nice extra step if you're feeling like you're a contestant on a competitive cooking show.

Chili powder heat varies, so taste the mole often while you're cooking. You can add a pinch of cayenne to up the heat without throwing the balance off and destroying the universe.

Buckwheat Waffles with Red Wine Tarragon Mushroom Gravy

Serves 6

Waffles are the perfect vehicle for sauce, with their little pockets ready and waiting. Reminiscent of the quintessential Russian dish buckwheat blini, this is one of my favorite ways to enjoy buckwheat waffles—absolutely smothered with rich, silky mushroom gravy.

Preheat a large pan over medium heat. Sauté the shallots in oil for 5 to 7 minutes, until lightly browned. Add the garlic and sauté for a minute more. Mix in the mushrooms, add pepper, and sauté for about 5 more minutes, until mushrooms are softened. Add the red wine and salt and turn heat up to high. Let wine reduce for about 5 minutes, stirring often.

Meanwhile, measure out the vegetable broth and mix in the flour. Stir well until few lumps are left. When the wine has reduced, lower the heat back to medium and pour in the vegetable broth mixture. Mix in the herbs. Stir often for about 15 more minutes; the gravy should be thick and creamy.

TO ASSEMBLE

For round waffles, cut into quarters and place on plate all pointing in the same direction. Pour gravy over the top and garnish with fresh thyme.

For the gravy:

2 tablespoons olive oil

1½ cups thinly sliced shallots

3 garlic cloves, minced

1 pound cremini mushrooms, thinly sliced

Several dashes black pepper

½ cup dry red cooking wine

½ teaspoon salt

2 cups cold vegetable broth

⅓ cup all-purpose flour

2 tablespoons chopped fresh tarragon

1 tablespoon chopped fresh thyme, plus additional for garnish

For serving:

1 recipe Buckwheat Waffles, savory variation (page 93)

Mom's Morning Casserole

Serves 8

My mom actually doesn't make a casserole like this, I was just inspired by those magazines at the supermarket checkout—the ones with recipes that begin with a thing of frozen hash browns and end with a tub of "processed cheese food." This casserole uses a bunch of mixing bowls but comes together easily and makes a flavorful and filling meal: a layer of paprika potatoes, a layer of scrambled tofu, and a layer of fennel-spiked tempeh and chopped red bell pepper, all topped off with some melted cheese. You can use your favorite cheeze sauce recipe in place of packaged vegan cheese or the Cheesy Sauce (page 217). This casserole makes a lot of food and tastes great at room temperature, making it a perfect potluck recipe. Serve with a salad or sautéed greens.

Make ahead: Bake potatoes and assemble casserole the night before. Let cool and wrap tightly in plastic wrap, store in the fridge overnight.

For the potato layer:

2 large yellow potatoes (about 1½ pounds)

1 tablespoon olive oil

2 teaspoons sweet paprika

½ teaspoon salt

For the tempeh layer:

1 pound tempeh

1 red bell pepper, seeded and finely chopped

2 garlic cloves, minced

2 tablespoons soy sauce

1 teaspoon olive oil

1 tablespoon fresh lemon juice (juice of ½ lemon)

1 teaspoon fennel seed, crushed

2 teaspoons dry rubbed sage (not powdered)

Fresh black pepper

Preheat the oven to 350°F. Slice the potatoes width-wise into ¼-inch-thick slices. You don't need to break out a ruler and measure them, but be careful to cut evenly and to not make them too thick or they won't cook through. Spread them out in an 11 x 13-inch baking pan to make sure that everything will fit (overlapping is necessary). Drizzle in the olive oil, add the paprika and salt, and use your hands to coat the potato slices. Then place them in overlapping layers to cover the bottom of the pan.

Bake for 25 minutes while you prepare the other layers. If you aren't done preparing the other layers by the time 25 minutes is up, that's okay, just remove potatoes from the oven and set aside until ready. The potatoes should be easily pierced with a fork; if they are not then bake for a few minutes more.

For the tofu layer:

2 pounds firm or extra-firm tofu

2 garlic cloves, minced

2 tablespoons soy sauce

2 teaspoons olive oil

1 tablespoon fresh lemon juice (juice of ½ lemon)

2 teaspoons ground cumin

2 tablespoons chopped fresh thyme (2 teaspoons if using dried)

½ teaspoon turmeric

Fresh black pepper

Salt, to taste

2 tablespoons nutritional yeast (optional)

For the topping:

½ pound shredded vegan cheese

MAKE THE TEMPEH LAYER

In a small mixing bowl, crumble the tempeh into pieces ranging in size from pea-size to popcorn-size. Add the remaining tempeh layer ingredients and mix together until tempeh is coated.

MAKE THE TOFU LAYER

Give the tofu a squeeze over the sink to release some of the water. Place in a medium-size mixing bowl and use a fork to mash the tofu into a ricotta consistency. Add the remaining tofu layer ingredients and mix well. Taste for salt.

Your potatoes should be done baking by now. Remove them from the oven. Spread the tofu over the potatoes and press it firmly into the pan with a spatula (careful, because the pan is still hot). Sprinkle the tempeh over the tofu and return pan to the oven. Bake for 20 minutes.

Remove the casserole from the oven and sprinkle the cheese over the top. Return it to the oven and bake for 10 more minutes. If the cheese hasn't melted, place in the broiler for a minute or two. If you're using a cheese sauce instead, then there's no need to remove the casserole from the oven after the first 20 minutes. Just bake for 30 minutes total and pour the cheese sauce over the top when done.

Let cool for about 10 minutes, slice into eight pieces, and serve.

TIP

Mince the garlic for both the tempeh and the tofu layers at the same time.

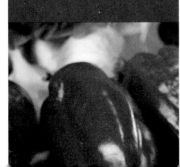

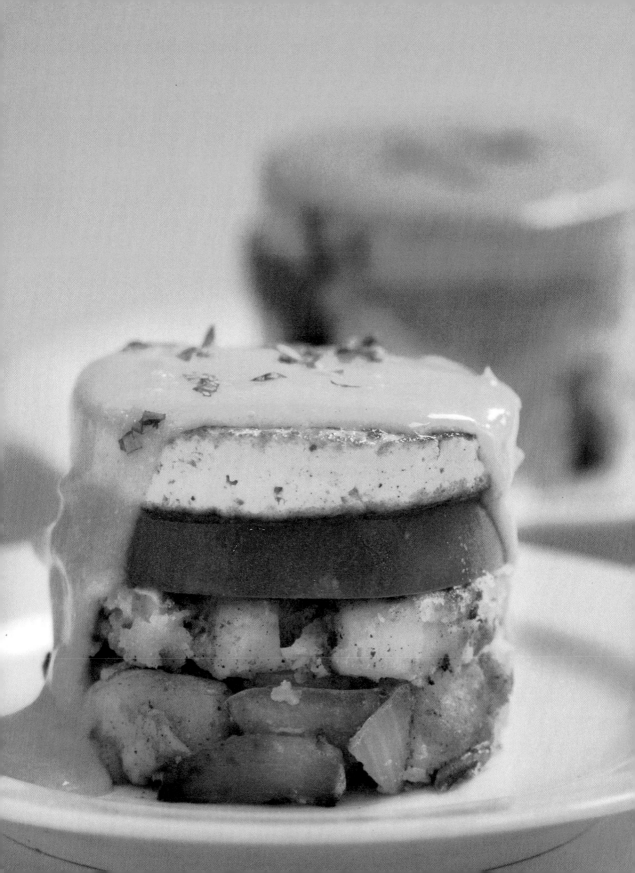

Tofu Benny

Serves 6

I crave Eggs Benedict—the tanginess, the smokiness—and this is my favorite vegan translation to date. Standing in for the ham this morning is a delicious juicy tomato, sprinkled with smoked salt. You might not have smoked salt lying around, and so I give you another option, even though I think you should run out and buy some. It's one of those ingredients that just ups the ante and makes such a difference, so take this opportunity to elevate your spice rack. The same goes for the black salt.

The recipe looks more fussy than it is, so don't let it scare you. It's really just a matter of marinating some tofu and making a sauce and some home fries.

Make ahead: You can marinate the tofu overnight.

PREPARE THE TOFU

Combine all the marinade ingredients in a large mixing bowl. Gently press some of the water out of the tofu. Lay the tofu on its narrow side and slice into three pieces lengthwise. So basically you will have three slices that are large, flat rectangles. Use a 3-inch cookie cutter to cut circles out of each tofu slice. Repeat with the next block of tofu. Reserve the rest of the tofu for another use, it will be about a pound of leftover (see the Garden Herb Spread recipe on page 210, which calls for exactly that amount).

2 pounds firm tofu

1 recipe Diner Home Fries (page 117) or 6 English Muffins (page 190)

1 recipe Hollandaise Sauce (page 218)

Chopped fresh herbs for garnish (thyme, chives, tarragon, parsley ... most anything will work)

For the marinade:

1 tablespoon soy sauce

½ teaspoon ground mustard

1 cup vegetable broth

¼ teaspoon arrowroot

1 teaspoon black salt

2 tablespoons white wine vinegar

2 tablespoons olive oil, plus more for cooking

For the tomatoes:

6 large slices beefsteak or heirloom tomato (any large, juicy tomato, really)

Smoked salt, to taste, or 1 teaspoon liquid smoke and a sprinkle of sea salt

Marinate the tofu circles for about an hour, but it's great to do overnight, too.

To time this right, you should start cooking the tofu when you're letting the hollandaise sauce cool (see Hollandaise Sauce directions, page 218). It's really simple, just preheat a cast-iron pan over medium heat, add a thin layer of olive oil and cook on each side till nicely browned, about 15 minutes total.

PREPARE THE PLATES

If using English muffins, just toast 'em and put 'em on down with their tops off to the side. If you're using home fries, it's cute to mold them into a ring. You can use a large round cookie cutter as the mold, just firmly pack the home fries into the ring, lift it, and voilà! A perfect mound of home fries. Or, if you'd rather, just plop the home fries down on the plate.

Now put a tomato on the English muffin or home fries. It's cool and fancy if the tomato slice is the same size as your base, but it doesn't matter that much. Sprinkle with a pinch of smoked salt, if using. Otherwise, drizzle with just a touch of liquid smoke (you can dab it on with your fingertips, just don't overdo it) and sprinkle with a little sea salt.

Next, place your tofu on the tomato. And last but not least, pour the hollandaise on top and sprinkle on your herb garnish. Now say something French; you deserve it!

TIP
I think it's really cute to cut the tofu into large circles. It makes for a fancier-looking dish. But if you don't want to do that, you can use just one block of firm tofu and cut it into eighths widthwise, then proceed with the rest of the recipe. I use firm tofu here, not extra-firm, because I like for the outside to be chewy and the inside just a bit creamy. Shoot for tomatoes that have a 3-inch circumference so that your Benny stacks nicely.

Chili Cashew Dosas with Spiced Apple Cider Chutney

Makes 14 dosas

Savory, lacy, and crispy, this South Indian–style treat is crammed with substantially flavorful nuts, onions, and spices, so it doesn't require the potato filling typically served with these super-thin crepes. The Spiced Apple Cider Chutney (page 72) makes for an offbeat and delightful fall or winter pancake brunch. These "rava"-style dosas are relatively petite compared to ones made in restaurants, but they deliver all the flavor and are fun to make when you get the hang of it.

If the idea of dosas at home makes you nervous, it's time to go the distance with your crepe-making skills (or build those skills if you don't have them yet). Just like with crepes, dosa practice makes dosa perfect, and surely your last batch will kick the butt of the first.

In a large bowl, stir together Cream of Wheat cereal, rice flour, chickpea flour, salt, pepper, and cumin seeds. Pour in 3½ cups water, stirring until no lumps remain. Set aside batter for at least ½ hour. Now would be a good time to prepare some chutney if using.

When ready to cook, stir in red onion, cashews, jalapeños, and ½ cup additional water. The batter

1 cup Cream of Wheat cereal, uncooked

½ cup rice flour

½ cup chickpea flour

2 teaspoons salt

½ generous teaspoon freshly cracked peppercorns (just grind whole peppercorns as coarsely as possible)

1½ teaspoons cumin seeds

3½ cups water, plus up to 1 cup extra

½ cup very finely chopped red onion

½ cup chopped, toasted cashews

1–2 jalapeños, seeded and chopped

Vegetable oil for frying (any kind that is well suited for higher temperatures, such as peanut or high-heat canola)

1 recipe Spiced Apple Cider Chutney (page 72)

should be very thin, almost alarmingly so, and even thinner than crepe batter. It will appear similar to thick soy milk. Keep handy at least ½ cup of additional water to thin out the batter if it should thicken during the cooking of dosas.

Preheat a crepe pan over medium-high heat. The pan is ready when a few droplets of water flicked onto the surface sizzle. Brush the pan generously with oil. Stir batter, scoop a ladle-full, and in an outward circular motion pour the batter onto the hot pan. The batter will sizzle, bubble, and fail to form a perfect circle, and that's okay! Gently tip the pan side to side to evenly distribute any excess batter. The dosa surface should have plenty of holes and be very thin; if it looks too thick, use less batter for the next one. If your dosas still appear too thick or doughy, try thinning out the batter even more with a little water, a few tablespoons at a time. Make sure to stir the batter each time before ladling it onto the pan.

Cook each dosa for about 2 to 3 minutes. As the top of the dosa starts to dry and the edges brown, use the silicon brush to dribble a little extra oil over the dosa. Use the long thin spatula to lift up the dosa's edges, then carefully run the spatula underneath to dislodge it completely from the pan. If your dosa is sticking, use more oil the for the next one. Carefully use the spatula to fold the dosa in half; cook for 1 minute, flip and cook for another minute. An alternate way of folding a rava-style dosa is to mentally divide your round dosa into thirds, and flip the edges of each third about a third of the way in toward the center. Your resulting round dosa has now been transformed into a triangle. Flip it over and cook it for another minute or so and you're done.

Move cooked dosas to a serving plate and eat immediately. Dosas are best eaten piping hot with your fingers. Rip off a bit and dip it into a sauce or chutney.

❋ VARIATION ❋

FRUIT AND NUT DOSAS

Omit jalapeño. Add ½ cup golden raisins to the flours and spices. Proceed as directed.

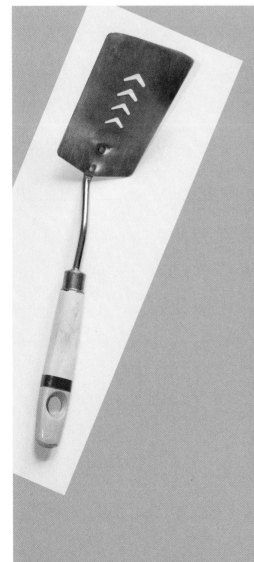

TIP The right tools make dosa cookery a breeze. A 10- to 12-inch crepe pan is the next-best thing to the huge round cooking griddles typically used for dosa making, but any well-seasoned cast-iron pan will do. If you must use nonstick cookware, be sure to use only silicon or rubber tools on it. You'll also need a heat-proof basting brush for spreading the oil (I like silicon brushes) and a long, thin metal spatula. The best kind for the job are the long ones often used for frosting cakes, bent near the handle and curved at the tip. Last but never least, a metal ladle (⅓ cup to ½ cup-size) for pouring the batter will be your friend in the journey of dosa nirvana.

Usually dosa batter is allowed to sit for a day or so to ferment and develop a deeper, slightly tangy flavor. For the sake of speed we ditched that part. But if you have the time, allow the batter (minus onions, jalapeños, and cashews) to sit covered on a countertop overnight. An hour before cooking, add onions, jalapeños, and cashews and continue as directed.

Spiced Apple Cider Chutney

Makes 2 cups

This chutney is completely American in character but made a tad Indian by the addition of mustard seeds. After pairing with dosas, use up the leftovers (if there are any) by serving with any fried or roasted potato dish. This chutney nicely complements bitter sautéed greens as well.

In a medium saucepan over medium heat combine oil and mustard seeds. Stir and cook mustard seeds till they start to pop, less than 1 minute. Add ginger and onion, stirring and cooking till onion begins to soften, about 3 to 4 minutes. Stir in the apples and cook for another 2 minutes, then pour in apple cider, raisins, spices, brown sugar, and vinegar. Increase the heat to bring the mixture to a boil. Stir, then reduce heat to low and cook for 25 to 30 minutes, until the apples are really soft and most of the liquid has evaporated. Allow to cool before serving and store in the fridge.

2 teaspoons vegetable oil

1 teaspoon mustard seeds

1-inch cube ginger, peeled and finely chopped

½ cup finely chopped sweet white onion, about 1 small onion

1 pound apples, cored and diced, about 2 large apples

1½ cups apple cider

½ cup golden raisins or finely chopped dates

½ teaspoon each ground cinnamon and nutmeg

3 tablespoons brown sugar

3 tablespoons apple cider vinegar

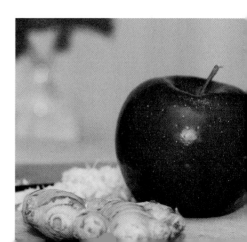

Courico Tacos with Grilled Pineapple Salsa

Makes 8 tacos

A chewy and, dare I say, *meaty*, spicy taco topped with sweet, caramelized Grilled Pineapple Salsa (page 76). I read about *courico* in just about every foodie magazine, blog, and book there is, so it got my attention. It's a Portuguese version of chorizo sausage, and it's supposed to be a little vinegary (apple cider vinegar) and a little sweet (a drop of sugar) and a little smoky (chipotle peppers). Red wine usually makes an appearance in these recipes, too.

I also read about soy curls in just about every vegan blog, and so I thought that the two phenomena should meet. If you can't find soy curls, then 2½ cups sliced seitan should do nicely. Obviously, in that case you would skip the step where you soak the curls and just add the seitan to the pan.

You can mail order the soy curls from Food Fight! Vegan Grocery (www.foodfightgrocery.com) or substitute seitan.

Put soy curls in a bowl and cover with warm water. Let sit for about 5 minutes, stirring occasionally so that they soak evenly. Drain in a colander and gently squeeze them to remove some of the water. If using seitan, just skip this step and cut the seitan into bite-size pieces.

To assemble:

8 taco shells, steamed, microwaved, or otherwise warmed up

For the courico:

2 cups soy curls or 1½ cups seitan

2 tablespoons olive oil

1 medium-size yellow onion, diced small

4 garlic cloves, minced

2 tablespoons soy sauce

2 to 6 chipotles in adobe sauce, seeds removed, chopped very thoroughly (almost pulverized)

2 tablespoons chopped fresh marjoram (or oregano), or 2 teaspoons dried

4 teaspoons ground cumin

2 teaspoons mild chili powder

½ teaspoon anise seed

½ teaspoon salt

½ cup red wine

1 tablespoon sugar

1 fifteen-ounce can stewed tomatoes

1 tablespoon apple cider vinegar

1 recipe Grilled Pineapple Salsa (page 76)

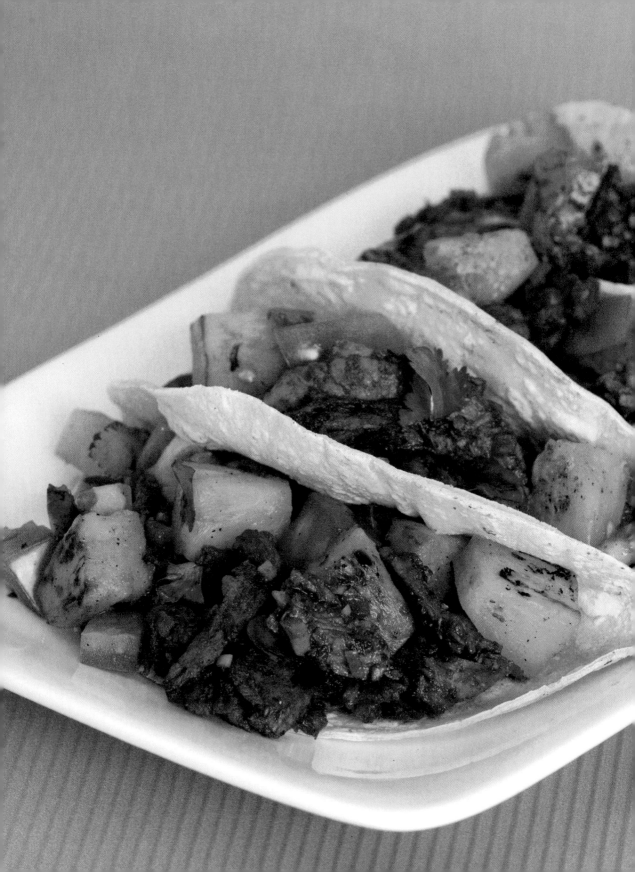

Preheat a large pan over medium heat. Sauté the onion in the oil for 5 to 7 minutes, until the onion is translucent. Add the garlic, sauté for about another minute. Add the soy curls and soy sauce, and turn the heat up. Cook for about 5 minutes on high heat, until soy curls get a little browned.

Add chipotles, marjoram, cumin, chili powder, anise seed, and salt. Sauté for another minute. Add the wine, sugar, tomatoes, and vinegar. Cook for 10 minutes or so on high heat, stirring occasionally, until most of the liquid is absorbed.

Let sit for at least 10 minutes before serving. The courico tastes better the longer it sits, so if you can make this dish an hour before you're ready to serve and then reheat, that would be ideal.

TO ASSEMBLE
You can figure this out, right?

Grilled
Pineapple Salsa

Preheat an outdoor grill or a cast-iron grill pan over high heat. Brush the pineapple with oil. Grill for 4 to 5 minutes on each side, until charred and a bit caramelized. Remove the pineapple from the grill and place on a plate to cool. Once cool enough to handle, cut the pineapple slices into ½-inch chunks.

Combine all ingredients well and chill until ready to use.

Vegetable oil for brushing

½ pineapple (about 1½ pounds), cut into ½-inch long slices

1 small red onion, finely diced

1 small tomato, diced small

¼ cup chopped cilantro

1 tablespoon lime juice

Ethiopian Crepes

Makes 8 crepes

Ethiopian food for breakfast? Oh, hell yes. The scents of curry and clove will warm up your kitchen. This recipe features my cheater Ethiopian spice blend. Although the spice list looks really long, it's usually twice that. Crepes are a great stand-in for the traditional and delicious but hard to make fermented bread called *injera* that is usually served with Ethiopian food. This is made to go with the Coleslaw Potato Salad with Cumin Seeds (page 120), a cool and creamy complement to this rich spicy stew. You will definitely have filling leftovers, so serve them with rice for dinner any night of the week. This makes 8 crepes, so you can serve either 1 or 2 to each diner depending on what else you are serving that morning.

First cook the lentils. Boil them in about 5 cups of water for half an hour or until tender. Drain and set aside.

Preheat a soup pot over medium heat. Sauté onion in olive oil for 5 to 7 minutes, until translucent. Add garlic and ginger, sauté another minute more. Add the spice blend and stir constantly for about a minute to toast the spices.

Add the tomatoes and lentils and simmer for about 15 minutes more. Let cool for about 15 minutes before assembling.

1 cup brown lentils

2 tablespoons olive oil

1 large onion, diced small

4 garlic cloves, minced

2 tablespoons fresh ginger, minced

1 twenty-four-ounce can crushed tomatoes

Spice blend:

2 teaspoons curry powder

2 teaspoons Hungarian paprika

2 teaspoons ground cumin

1 teaspoon dried thyme

¼ teaspoon ground cinnamon

¼ teaspoon ground cardamom

⅛ teaspoon ground allspice

⅛ teaspoon ground cloves

⅛ teaspoon cayenne

½ teaspoon salt, or to taste

8 Classic Crepes, **savory variation** (page 104)

1 recipe Coleslaw Potato Salad with Cumin Seeds (page 120)

Chopped fresh mint for garnish

TO ASSEMBLE

Spoon about ⅓ cup of stew onto the bottom third of the crepe. Fold bottom over filling and roll crepe up. If you're feeling adventurous, slice in half and serve over potato salad. Otherwise, just place on a plate with some salad on the side. Garnish with chopped fresh mint.

The Sweet

Pancakes, Waffles, French Toast, and Anything That Will Have You Licking Syrup from Your Plate

Banana Flapjacks

Makes 6 six-inch flapjacks

I'm trying to bring back the word "flapjacks"; how am I doing? These are big, fluffy pancakes with just a hint of spice that are perfect for cuddling up to. I use a ⅓-cup measuring cup for pouring them—I like 'em big rather than silver dollar–size. You can, of course, add any of the additions I've listed, but I find that they're perfect as is. Serve with plenty of maple syrup and margarine. For best results, use bananas that are very ripe and heavily spotted.

2 very ripe medium bananas

2 tablespoons canola oil

½ cup almond milk (or your favorite nondairy milk)

½ cup water

2 teaspoons apple cider vinegar

1 tablespoon pure maple syrup

1 cup all-purpose flour

2¼ teaspoons baking powder

¼ teaspoon salt

¼ teaspoon ground cinnamon (optional)

Pinch ground allspice (optional)

Cooking spray

Use a fork to mash bananas in a large mixing bowl. Add the oil, milk, water, vinegar, and maple syrup and mix well. Add the flour, baking powder, salt, and spices. Mix until there are very few clumps left. As usual, be careful not to overmix.

Preheat a large, heavy-bottomed, nonstick skillet (cast iron preferred) over medium heat for at least 3 minutes. You'll know the pan is hot enough by adding a drop of water—the water should dance around the pan, but the pan should not be smoking.

Spray the pan with a light coat of cooking spray (or a very light coat of oil). Pour pancakes one at a time in ½ cup measurements and cook until the top looks somewhat dry (about 3 minutes). Flip over and cook for another minute.

Transfer to a plate covered with tinfoil to keep the flapjacks warm while you prepare the others.

⁂ VARIATIONS ⁂

Fold in 1 cup chopped of any of the following: fresh berries, chocolate chips, shredded coconut, nuts.

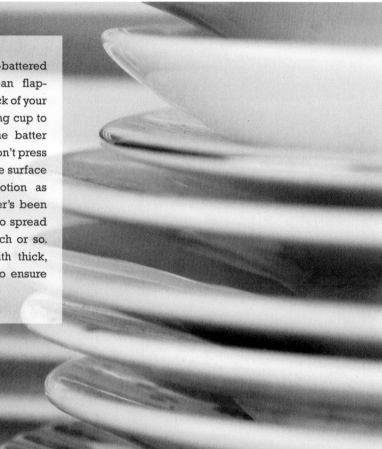

TIP For thick-battered pancakes (I mean flap-jacks) use the back of your ladle or measuring cup to gently spread the batter on the griddle. Don't press hard, just skim the surface in a circular motion as soon as the batter's been poured to get it to spread out by half an inch or so. It works well with thick, large pancakes to ensure even heating.

Gluten-Free Buckwheat Pancakes

Makes 8 four- to five-inch pancakes

Whether you're allergic to wheat, giving your tummy a rest, or just want to experiment with tasty and nutritious flours, these pancakes belong at your brunch table. They're light, airy, and really perfect for absorbing lots of maple syrup. Unless you have a gluten allergy, you may not have all these flours sitting around. You can play around with this recipe's flour ratios pretty interchangeably, so if you need to use all corn flour or all quinoa flour that's okay.

In a large mixing bowl, mix together all flours and the flax seeds, baking powder, cinnamon, and salt. Create a well in the center and add the remaining wet ingredients. Use a fork to mix well for about a minute. Let the batter rest for about 10 minutes and preheat a large, heavy-bottomed, nonstick pan, preferably cast iron, over medium-high heat.

When pan is hot, spray with a thin layer of cooking spray and use an ice cream scooper to pour batter and form pancakes. I usually make two at a time, but do as many as you can fit. The pancake should start to form little air bubbles, but not as much as "normal" pancakes do, so don't worry. Cook on one side for 2½ to 3 minutes, then flip and cook for 2 minutes more.

½ cup buckwheat flour

¼ cup quinoa flour

¼ cup corn flour (*not* cornmeal; corn flour is finer)

2 tablespoons tapioca flour (cornstarch or arrowroot would be okay, too)

1 tablespoon ground flax seeds (or flax meal)

1 tablespoon baking powder

¼ teaspoon cinnamon

¼ teaspoon salt

½ cup soy milk (or other nondairy milk)

½ cup water

2 tablespoons pure maple syrup

2 tablespoons canola oil

½ teaspoon pure vanilla extract

Cooking spray

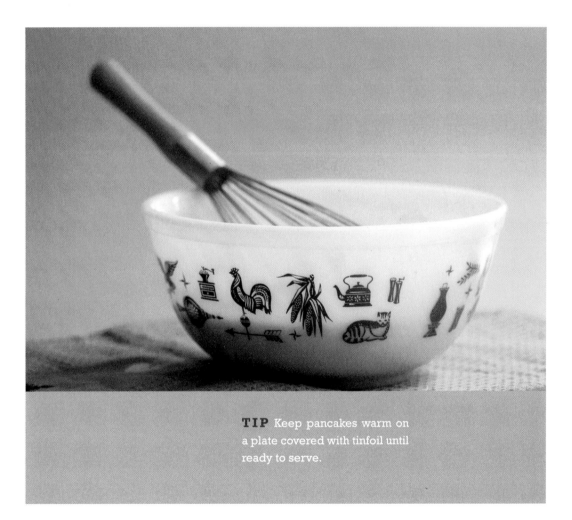

TIP Keep pancakes warm on a plate covered with tinfoil until ready to serve.

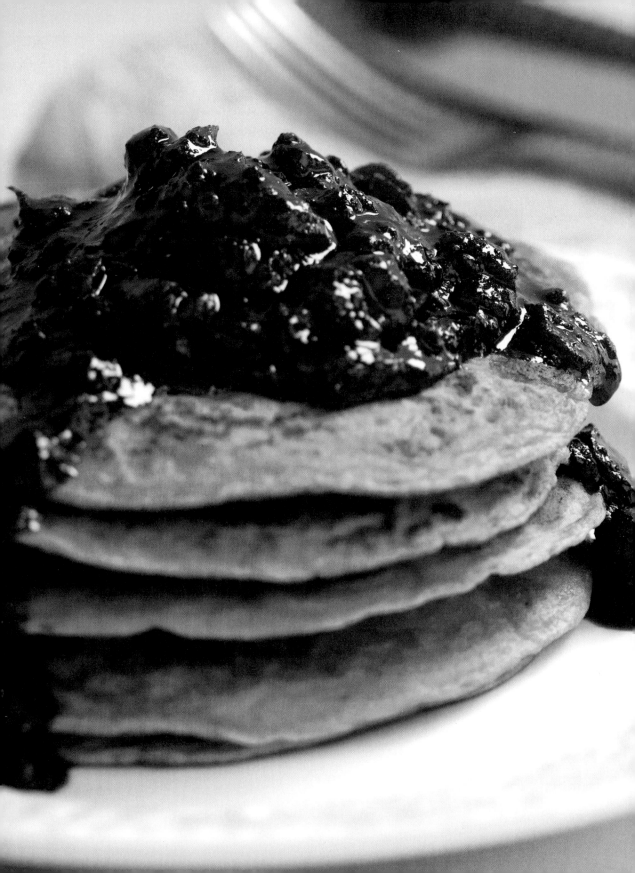

Pumpkin Pancakes

Makes 6 six-inch pancakes

Cinnamon and ginger really let pumpkin flaunt its flavor in this cheerfully orange pancake. These are a natural choice for Thanksgiving brunch, topped with Ginger Cranberry Sauce (page 200). But there's no law against enjoying them any time of year.

In a large mixing bowl, whisk together pumpkin, oil, milk, water, vinegar, maple syrup, and vanilla. Add the flour, baking powder, salt, and spices. Mix until there are very few clumps left. As usual, be careful not to overmix.

Preheat a large, heavy-bottomed, nonstick skillet (cast iron preferred) over medium heat for at least 3 minutes. You'll know the pan is hot enough by adding a drop of water—the water should dance around the pan, but the pan should not be smoking.

Spray the pan with a light coat of cooking spray (or a very light coat of oil). Pour pancakes in ½ cup measurements, one at a time, and cook until the top looks somewhat dry (about 3 minutes). Flip over and cook for another minute.

Transfer to a plate covered with tinfoil to keep pancakes warm while you prepare the others.

¾ cup pureed or canned pumpkin

2 tablespoons canola oil

¾ cup almond milk (any nondairy milk will do)

½ cup water

2 teaspoons apple cider vinegar

2 tablespoons pure maple syrup

1 teaspoon pure vanilla extract

1 cup all-purpose flour

2 teaspoons baking powder

½ teaspoon salt

1 teaspoon ground cinnamon

1 teaspoon ground ginger

¼ teaspoon ground nutmeg

Pinch ground cloves

Cooking spray

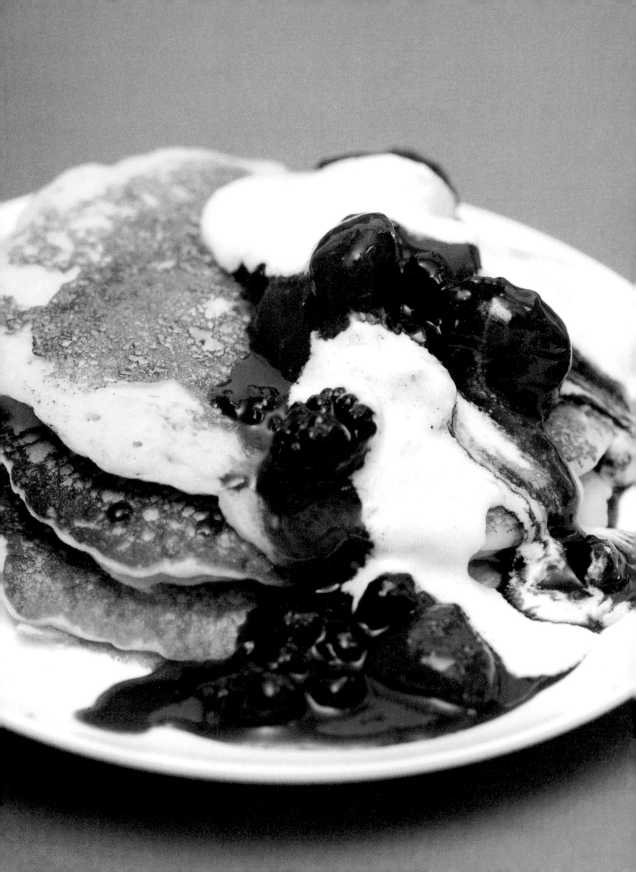

Perfect Pancakes

Makes 8 four- to five-inch pancakes

There's no greater comfort then tucking into a stack of pancakes dripping with syrup and piled high with strawberries and bananas. When I first went vegan as a teenager I remember going to my neighborhood diner with some friends for some midnight pancakes, coffee, and doing stupid stuff with those little half-and-half containers. Being the lone vegan at the table I had to watch *Clockwork Orange*–style as my friends devoured pancake after pancake while I picked at my dry bagel. When I got home I immediately made my own pancakes and ate them 'til the sun came up. Who needs sleep when you're 17?

This recipe was originally published in *Vegan with a Vengeance*, but I would be remiss not to include it here. So think of it as a bonus, not as some sort of scam to get you to buy recipes that you may already have.

1¼ cups all-purpose flour

2 teaspoons baking powder

½ teaspoon salt

1 teaspoon ground cinnamon (optional)

2 tablespoons canola oil

⅓ cup water

1 to 1¼ cups plain rice milk or soy milk

2 tablespoons pure maple syrup

1 teaspoon pure vanilla extract

Cooking spray

Preheat a large skillet over medium heat for at least 2 minutes (and up to 5 minutes).

In a large bowl, sift together the flour, baking powder, salt, and cinnamon. Make a well in the center and add the oil, water, milk, maple syrup, and vanilla. Mix just until ingredients are combined. A few lumps in the batter are just fine.

Spray the pan with a light coat of cooking spray (or a very light coat of oil). Pour pancakes one at a time and cook until bubbles form and the top looks somewhat dry (about 3 minutes). Flip over and cook for another minute. Serve!

Old-Fashioned Chelsea Waffles

Makes 4 six-inch round waffles or 8 four-inch square ones

When my brother and I were kids we would go to this diner in Chelsea for waffles. We'd have them with way too much syrup and a black-and-white egg cream and sit and watch all the Manhattan people rushing by. We were only 10 years old but my dad thought it was totally acceptable to send us to a NYC diner all alone, still dressed in our pajamas.

Anyway, the waffles there had a malted, toasty taste that I loved, crispy outside and more tender inside. In this recipe I used a little barley malt syrup and some cornmeal to achieve those flavors and textures, respectively. If you don't want to get the barley malt syrup, just use maple syrup instead. The waffles will taste a little sweeter but still totally good.

2 cups almond milk (or your favorite nondairy milk)

1 teaspoon apple cider vinegar

3 tablespoons canola oil

3 tablespoons barley malt syrup (at room temperature)

1¾ cups all-purpose flour

¼ cup cornmeal

½ teaspoon salt

1 tablespoon baking powder

1 tablespoon cornstarch

Cooking spray

Preheat your waffle iron.

In a large mixing bowl use a fork to vigorously mix together milk, vinegar, oil, and barley malt syrup, until barley malt syrup is dissolved.

Add remaining dry ingredients and mix together until the batter is smooth. Spray the waffle iron with cooking spray and cook waffles according to manufacturer's directions.

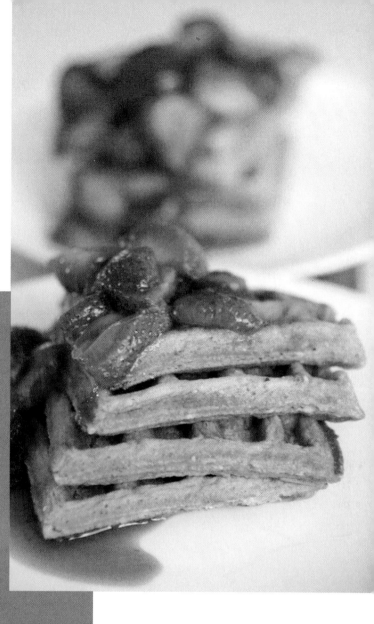

Leggo My Eggoless Waffle

Freezing waffles is a great brunch strategy for myriad reasons. First off, you can make them a few days in advance so that you have time to do other things on the day of a large brunch—like try to find vodka for your Bloody Marys at 8 in the morning.

There is also a benefit to toasting frozen waffles: it crisps the outside nicely. This is especially helpful if you have a rinky-dink waffle iron that doesn't quite do the crisping job as well as you like.

And even if you're not doing brunch, a batch of waffles in the fridge is great for weekday breakfasts. You can even eat them walking down the street, with a bunch of bananas stuffed in between or a few spoonfuls of your favorite jam.

To reheat waffles, just toast for about 3 minutes. Meanwhile, lean against the counter and think about how smart and efficient you are.

Peanut Butter Waffles

Makes 4 six-inch round waffles or 6 four-inch square ones

When faced with figuring out a way to fit peanut butter into brunch, these waffles become the obvious choice. Use chunky peanut butter for the most intense peanut-ty taste. The batter is really thick and also very forgiving—you can use practically any flour and they still come out great! But don't go trying that with every recipe; these are special.

Preheat your waffle iron. In a large mixing bowl, mix together peanut butter, maple syrup, and canola oil until well combined. Separately, mix together the milk and cornstarch in a measuring cup and add to the batter along with the vanilla.

Add flour, baking powder, salt, and nutmeg and mix until the batter is relatively smooth.

Spray the waffle iron with cooking spray and cook waffles according to manufacturer's directions.

¾ cup chunky natural peanut butter

3 tablespoons pure maple syrup

3 tablespoons canola oil

2 cups soy milk

1 tablespoon cornstarch

1 teaspoon pure vanilla extract

2¼ cups white whole wheat flour (all-purpose or whole wheat pastry flour work, too)

1 tablespoon baking powder

¾ teaspoon salt

¼ teaspoon ground nutmeg (use fresh grated if you can)

Cooking spray

The Waffle Truth

I remember the first time someone told me they made their own waffles. I was shocked. I was dismissive. I remember asking, "But are they good?" I just couldn't believe that something requiring such complicated machinery was within my reach. And once I tried it myself I was addicted. Don't make the same mistake I did and waste your life being intimidated by a gadget—dive in with a waffle maker. Here are a few tips I've picked up along the way.

1. Just following orders—read your waffle maker directions

Waffle irons differ so drastically from iron to iron that I can't give directions for the actual waffle-making process, so I just end each recipe with "cook waffles according to manufacturer's directions." But generally you grease the iron, pour the batter in, and close the lid. You know it's ready when the light either goes off or comes on, depending on your waffle maker. A general rule of thumb is that when the waffle stops steaming you know it's done. Remember to always give your iron plenty of time to heat up and to grease it between every waffle, no exceptions. That gets you a nice crispy outside.

2. Love will tear us apart—and our waffles

It happens to the best of us. You smell all that waffle-y goodness, lift the lid, and … OUCH! The top of the waffle rips right off, revealing the soft, delicate, and now useless insides. There are a few reasons this might happen. Numero uno is that the waffle wasn't done cooking. If you have a heat dial on your iron, turn it down a bit, so that the outside won't cook way before the inside. Another culprit might be a batter that is too thick. Add a few tablespoons of liquid and see if that helps the next one. And did you remember to grease the waffle iron between every waffle?

3. You should only be able to see through the waffle if you're Superman

Yes, unless you have X-ray vision, your waffle shouldn't be transparent or have any holes in it. This means your batter was way too thin. Add a few tablespoons of flour and try again!

4. Too much of a good thing—don't overfill your waffle iron

Use a measuring cup to pour your batter so that you know how much is the right amount for your iron. Overfilling can lead to many a waffle crime such as rippages (see above), raw or undercooked sides, and just big fat messes. Usually a scant one cup of batter is good for a 6-inch waffle iron.

5. To spread or not to spread?

I say don't try to spread the batter out. Just drop it into the center of the iron and let the waffle iron do the work. Once you close the lid the batter will spread out all on its own.

Of course, it sucks to waste waffle batter and it's nice to know if you're in for any trouble before you begin cooking. If you're feeling super-paranoid, or you're working with a new waffle iron, you can do a test. Just pour 2 tablespoons of batter into the iron and make a little mini-waffle to see how it comes out.

Cornbread Waffles

Makes 6 six-inch round waffles or 8 four-inch square ones

Who can resist cornbread in the morning? These waffles are nice and dense yet somehow still light and airy. It sounds impossible but try them and see. For savory waffles, just reduce the sugar by two tablespoons.

Preheat your waffle iron. Measure out the milk in a large measuring cup and add the vinegar to it. Set mixture aside to curdle.

In a large mixing bowl, mix together cornmeal, flour, baking powder, salt, and sugar. Make a well in the center and add the milk mixture and oil. Mix together until relatively smooth. Spray the waffle iron with cooking spray and cook waffles according to manufacturer's directions.

2 cups almond milk (or your favorite nondairy milk)

1 teaspoon apple cider vinegar

1½ cups cornmeal

1 cup all-purpose flour

1 tablespoon baking powder

½ teaspoon salt

¼ cup sugar (or 2 tablespoons sugar if making savory waffles)

¼ cup canola oil

Cooking spray

Buckwheat Waffles

Makes 6 six-inch round waffles or 8 four-inch square ones

Buckwheat has a distinctively nutty taste. Whenever I cook with it, the kitchen smells so pleasantly warm and homey, it makes me feel like I'm back in Mother Russia and getting a big hug from my grandma. Or at a really swank brunch joint on the Lower East Side getting pissed off at all the supermodels surrounding me and the tiny chairs that only fit half my butt.

Measure out the milk and water and add the vinegar to it. Set aside to curdle.

In a large mixing bowl, mix together buckwheat, flour, baking powder, salt, and sugar. Make a well in the center and add the milk mixture and oil. Mix together until relatively smooth. Let batter rest for 10 minutes. Meanwhile, preheat your waffle iron.

Spray the waffle iron with cooking spray and cook waffles according to manufacturer's directions.

1 cup almond milk (or nondairy milk of your choice)

1 cup water

2 teaspoons apple cider vinegar

¾ cup buckwheat flour

¾ cup all-purpose flour

1 teaspoon baking powder

½ teaspoon salt

3 tablespoons sugar (for savory waffles, reduce to 1 teaspoon)

¼ cup oil

Cooking spray

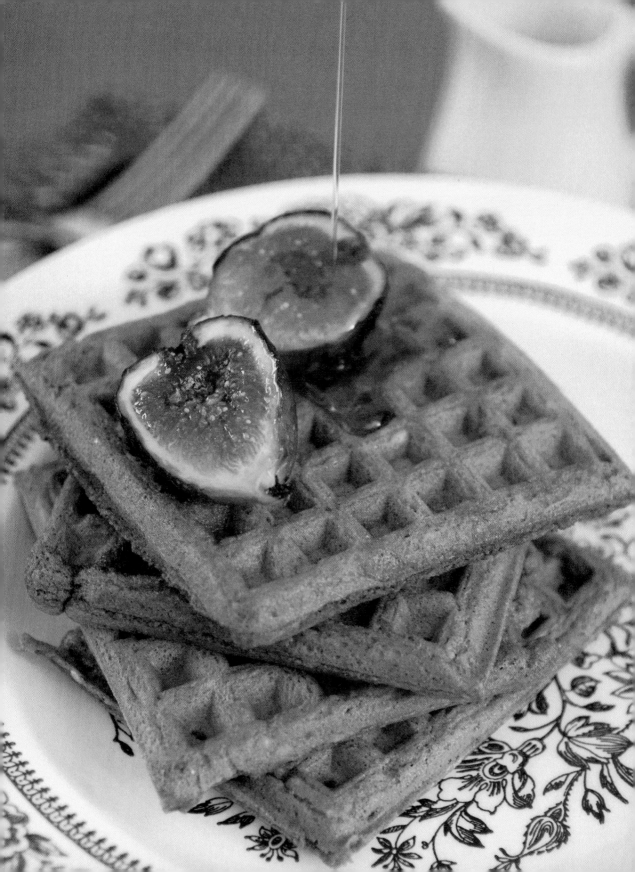

Gingerbread Waffles

Makes 4 six-inch round waffles or 8 four-inch square ones

The warming scents of ginger, cinnamon, and cloves will have you standing before your waffle iron absolutely drooling in anticipation. These are the perfect waffles for Christmas morning, even if you're Jewish. *That's* how good they are. Serve with caramelized figs for even more wintery perfection.

Preheat your waffle iron.

In a large mixing bowl use a fork to vigorously mix together milk, vinegar, oil, molasses, brown sugar, and vanilla. Mix until the molasses is mostly dissolved. Mix in the grated ginger.

Add remaining dry ingredients and mix together until smooth. Spray the waffle iron with cooking spray and cook waffles according to manufacturer's directions.

2 cups almond milk (or your favorite nondairy milk)

1 teaspoon apple cider vinegar

3 tablespoons canola oil

¼ cup molasses

½ cup brown sugar

1 teaspoon pure vanilla extract

2-inch knob ginger, peeled and grated (about 3 tablespoons)

2¼ cup all-purpose flour

½ teaspoon salt

2 teaspoons baking powder

1½ teaspoons cinnamon

¼ teaspoon ground cloves

Cooking spray

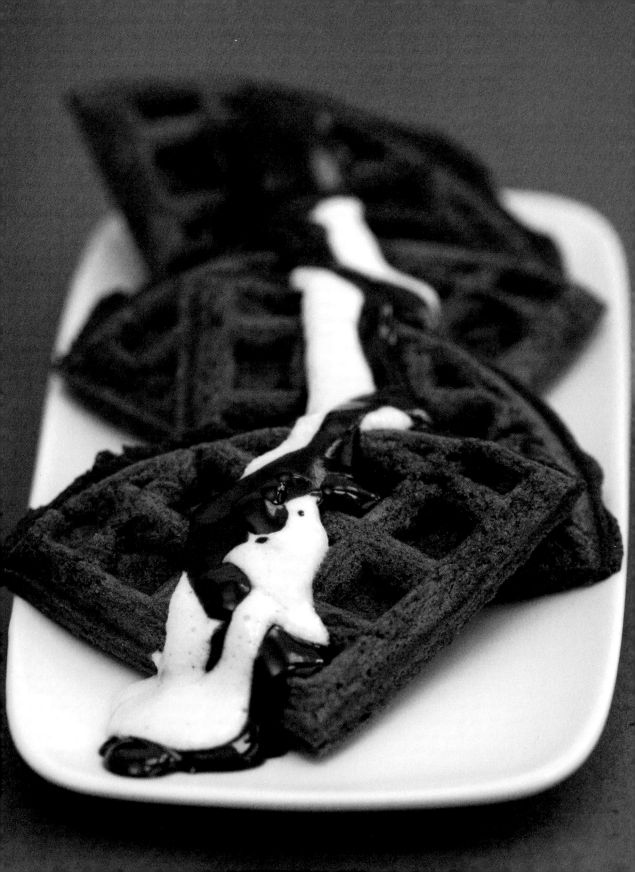

Chocolate Beer Waffles

Makes 6 six-inch round waffles or 8 four-inch square ones

You know how when you wake up the first thing you do is grab a chocolate bar and down a beer? Okay, well not you. Beer is a great cheerleader of chocolate. It boosts the flavor and gives these waffles a nice, silky texture. They are a real treat when topped with Chocolate Drizzle (page 208) and Sweet Cashew Cream (page 209). Yes, they are inching dangerously close to dessert, but …

Preheat your waffle iron. In a large mixing bowl, sift together flour, cocoa powder, baking powder, salt, and sugar.

Make a well in the center and add milk, beer, oil, and vanilla. Mix together until combined.

Spray the waffle iron with cooking spray and cook waffles according to manufacturer's directions. Serve with Chocolate Drizzle and Sweet Cashew Cream.

1 1/3 cups all-purpose flour

1/3 cup unsweetened cocoa powder

2 teaspoons baking powder

1/2 teaspoon salt

1/2 cup sugar

1 cup almond milk

3/4 cup porter, or other dark beer

1/4 cup canola oil

1 teaspoon pure vanilla extract

Cooking spray

Raised Waffles

Makes 6 six-inch round waffles or 8 four-inch square ones

Before we had the convenience of baking powder, our baked goods relied solely on yeast for their leavening. But besides just raising the waffles, yeast imparts a delicate and complex flavor. It's the perfect reason to break out your *Little House on the Prairie* DVDs and have a couple of friends from town over for a nice, old-fashioned breakfast with Ma and Pa.

If your waffle iron is capable of multiple settings, bake these at a higher temperature than usual so that they're crispy on the outside.

You have two choices for raising your batter: a single rise that takes about an hour, or let it rise for about half an hour at room temperature, then let it sit overnight in the refrigerator. The second way will give you a deeper yeasty flavor that is delicious.

2 cups warm almond milk (or your favorite nondairy milk)

2 teaspoons dry active yeast

¼ cup sugar

⅓ cup oil

1 teaspoon pure vanilla extract

2 cups all-purpose flour

¼ cup warm water

¾ teaspoon salt

Cooking spray

Pour the milk into a large mixing bowl. Make it a glass or ceramic one, because metal affects the yeast. And keep in mind that the batter will double in size after rising. Sprinkle in the yeast and let it dissolve for about 5 minutes.

Mix in the sugar, oil, and vanilla, then add in the flour. Stir until the batter is relatively smooth. Add the water to activate the yeast.

Cover with a damp cloth and let batter rise in a warm place for about an hour. Or let rise for half an hour, then place in the refrigerator and let sit overnight.

Preheat your waffle iron and mix the salt into the batter. Let batter rest while the iron heats up. Spray the waffle iron with cooking spray and cook waffles according to manufacturer's directions.

❈ VARIATIONS ❈

PECANS

Add **1½ cups very finely chopped pecans** to the batter after rising.

BLUEBERRIES

Fold **2 cups fresh or frozen blueberries** into the batter after rising.

STRAWBERRIES

Fold **2 cups chopped fresh strawberries** into the batter after rising.

APPLE CINNAMON

Mix **1 tablespoon ground cinnamon** into the dry ingredients, fold **2 cups finely diced apples** into the batter after rising.

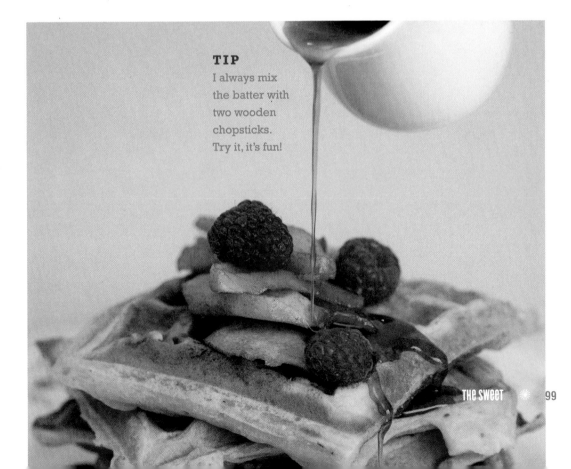

TIP
I always mix
the batter with
two wooden
chopsticks.
Try it, it's fun!

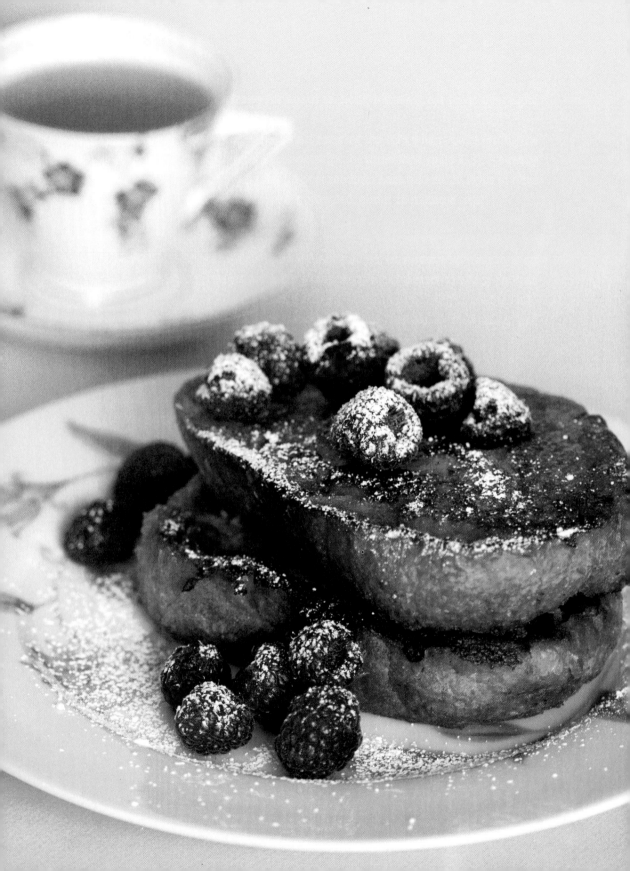

Pumpkin French Toast

Serves 4

During those crisp months of autumn I want pumpkin morning, noon, and night. This is a perfect way to use pureed pumpkin and pumpkin's favorite spices—cinnamon, ginger, and cloves.

Mix together pumpkin, milk, cornstarch, spices, and vanilla. Spread out sourdough slices on a rimmed baking pan in a single layer. Pour the pumpkin mixture onto the bread and flip slices to coat. Let sit for 10 minutes, then flip over and let soak for 10 minutes more.

Preheat a large, nonstick skillet (cast iron if you have it) over medium heat. Spray with cooking oil or drizzle a little oil into the pan. Cook about half the soaked bread for 5 to 7 minutes on one side and about 3 minutes on the other. When ready, the toast should be golden to medium brown and flecked with some darker spots. Keep warm on a plate covered with tinfoil while you cook the second batch.

If not serving immediately, cover the toast and place in a 200°F oven for up to an hour. Serve with maple syrup and margarine, of course.

1 cup pureed pumpkin (canned is just fine)

1½ cups almond milk (or your favorite nondairy milk)

2 tablespoons cornstarch

2 teaspoons cinnamon

1½ teaspoons ground ginger

½ teaspoon ground cloves

1 teaspoon pure vanilla extract

8 slices sourdough sliced in 1-inch-thick pieces

Cooking oil or cooking spray for the pan

TIP These French Toast recipes call for stale bread because it's going to be soaking up custard, but you still want the bread to hold its shape. Fresh bread will get mushy and, worst case scenario, fall apart. A three-day-old loaf should be just fine, while five days old might be too late (make it into breadcrumbs instead). If you have only a fresh loaf, you can cut the slices and then put them in a 300°F oven for about 10 minutes, until they are slightly hardened but not browned. Then proceed with the recipe.

Banana Rabanada (Brazilian French Toast)

Serves 4

Rabanada is a traditional Brazilian Christmas dish, but mark my words, you'll be craving it every weekend. A thickly sliced baguette is soaked in banana custard and panfried, then dusted all over with cocoa powder and cinnamon. Make sure to dust not just the baguette slices but the plate, too, so that the cocoa and cinnamon dissolve into the drippy syrup and you can sop it all up with each forkful. This recipe is quick and easy, but the bread does need 20 minutes to soak in the custard, so keep that in mind when planning your brunch.

Blend bananas, milk, cornstarch, and vanilla in a blender or food processor until smooth. Spread out baguette slices in a single layer on a baking pan. Pour banana mixture onto the bread and flip slices to coat. Let sit for 10 minutes, then flip over and let soak for 10 minutes more.

Preheat a large, nonstick skillet (cast iron preferred) over medium heat. Spray with cooking spray and cook about half of the soaked bread for 5 to 7 minutes on one side and about 3 minutes on the other. When ready, the toast should be golden to medium brown and flecked with darker spots. Keep warm on a plate covered with tinfoil while you cook the second batch.

2 very ripe bananas

1½ cups almond milk (or your favorite nondairy milk)

2 tablespoons cornstarch

1 teaspoon pure vanilla extract

1 tablespoon unsweetened cocoa powder

1 teaspoon ground cinnamon

1 stale baguette, sliced diagonally in 1-inch pieces (see Tip on page 101)

Cooking spray

Sliced strawberries and bananas for garnish

If not serving immediately, cover the toast with tinfoil and place in a 200°F oven for up to an hour.

When ready to serve, mix together cocoa powder and cinnamon and use a small sifter to sprinkle generously over each serving. Serve Rabanada with vegan butter and maple syrup, and topped with fresh fruit.

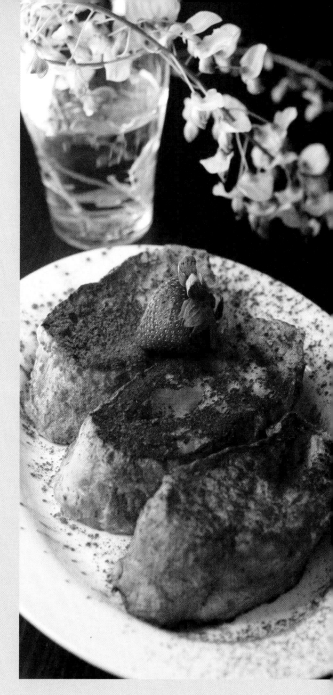

Crepes

Makes 10 to 12 crepes

The following recipes produce light and delicate crepes. You can serve them in so many ways: stuffed with bananas and zigzagged with Chocolate Drizzle (page 208) or stuffed with one of the fruit fillings of your choice. You can also just fold them up, sprinkle on powdered sugar, and serve with lemon wedges and maple syrup. Or, get a little fancier and try the sweet Lemon Cashew–Stuffed Crepes (page 108). Crepe making can be intimidating at first, but just follow the directions and read my Letter to a Young Crepe Maker (page 106) and you'll get the hang of it. It can be really helpful to see someone else make a crepe, so visit our Web site (www.theppk.com/shows) and watch Terry and me make crepes or just do a Google search for crepe making videos.

Put all the ingredients into a food processor or blender. Blend for about 30 seconds, scraping the sides of the blender once, until everything is smooth. The batter will be very thin. Refrigerate batter for about an hour. I just put the whole blender container in the fridge.

Preheat a crepe pan or large, nonstick skillet over medium-high heat. The pan is ready when a few drops of water flicked onto it sizzle. Lightly spray the pan with oil.

Ladle about ⅓ to ½ cup of batter (use the bigger amount for a bigger pan) in the center of the pan. Lift

Whole Wheat Crepes

1 cup almond milk (or your favorite nondairy milk)

1 cup water

1½ cups whole wheat pastry flour

2 tablespoons tapioca flour

1 teaspoon salt

2 tablespoons vegetable oil

2 tablespoons agave nectar or pure maple syrup

Classic Crepes

1½ cups almond milk (or your favorite nondairy milk)

¼ cup water

2 tablespoons agave nectar or pure maple syrup

¾ cup all-purpose flour

¼ cup chickpea flour

1 tablespoon tapioca flour (cornstarch or arrowroot is okay, too)

½ teaspoon salt

Cooking spray

the pan off the burner and tilt in a circular motion so that the batter spreads in a thin layer across the bottom.

Cook until the top of the crepe is dry, the center is bubbling, and the edges are lightly browned and crinkly and are pulling away from the sides of the pan, usually about 1 to 1½ minutes. Gently run the spatula under the crepe to loosen, then carefully flip and cook on the other side for 30 seconds. Slide the crepe onto a dinner plate. Repeat with the remaining crepes.

❋ VARIATION ❋

For savory crepes, as in the Ethiopian Crepes (page 77), just leave the agave out of the recipe.

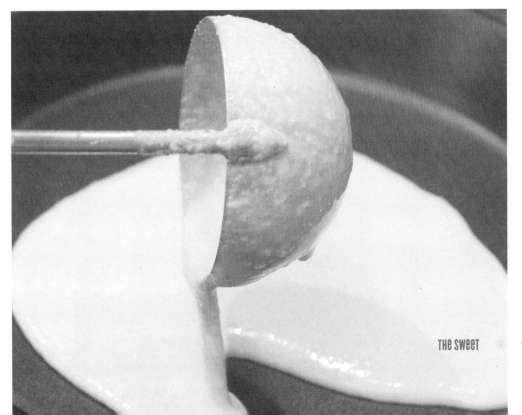

A Letter to a Young Crepe Maker

When I first started making crepes I found myself saying things like "don't panic," "it's okay," and "we'll get through this." Looking back, I don't see why crepes were so daunting. I suppose with anything delicate you're worried about breaking it. But one consolation is that messing up a crepe can be pretty entertaining. Like when you're tilting the pan to coat the bottom and the whole shebang slides right outta the pan and onto your cat.

The thing is, like so much in life, the anticipatory anxiety of crepe making is much worse than the actual process. I won't lie to you, you probably will ruin a crepe or two. It might tear, it might come out with an amoeba-like unevenness. But how will you know if you don't even try? And so what if you have a failed crepe? It doesn't make you a failed person. What does make you a failed person is failing to ever try making a crepe.

That said, there are some rules of engagement before entering the battlefield. These tips will minimize harm and hopefully save your cat from becoming an unwitting part of your brunch spread.

First things first, and that first thing is a crepe pan. Now, I am not going to say that you have to have one. But I am going to strongly imply it. The great thing about having a specific tool to do the job is that it is the perfect size and weight for tilting and the sides are sloped and curved just so. But if you're a beginner you probably don't have one—why would you? So choose the most lightweight and non-stick pan you've got. Once you find your true calling in life (crepe making, of course), invest in the pan.

Other tools you'll need are a super-thin and flexible spatula, preferably one that won't scrape your pan, and a ladle or measuring cup with which you can get consistently sized crepes. That is to say, don't pour the batter directly out of a container; always carefully measure it first.

Crepe batter is supposed to be thin. Much thinner than pancake batter. It should slide around easily as you pour it into the pan and tilt and swirl. You'll get better at gauging the right consistency for the batter as you get practice. But if your crepe is coming out like a pancake, add more water by the tablespoon until it starts to cooperate.

If your crepe is tearing when you try to flip it, just give it a little more time to cook or up the heat a bit. What you're looking for is a smooth, dry top, possibly with a few bubbles. The edges should appear paper thin and crinkly. If you shake the pan, the crepe should slide around without much coercion.

You can make crepes in advance, if you like. Just stack them up with a piece of wax paper in between each one and refrigerate. To reheat, simply heat your crepe pan, brush with a little margarine or a spray of nonstick cooking spray, and cook crepes for about 30 seconds each side.

But most importantly, get out there and make it happen. Those crepes won't make themselves. Yet.

Lemon Cashew–Stuffed Crepes with Whole Berry Sauce

Serves 4

This filling is akin to a sweet ricotta with a nice hint of lemon. Paired with Whole Berry Sauce (page 202), it makes a luscious crepe that almost seems like having cheesecake for breakfast. You need to soak the cashews overnight, so plan accordingly! I would advise making the berry sauce and the cashew filling first, and making the crepes last.

Make ahead: The cashews need to be soaked for at least 8 hours, so keep that in mind when planning this recipe. You can also make the entire filling a day ahead and refrigerate in a tightly sealed container.

MAKE THE LEMON CASHEW FILLING

In a mixing bowl, soak the cashews in water. Cover with plastic wrap and refrigerate overnight or at least 8 hours.

Drain cashews and add them to the food processor. Pulse a few times to break them up. Add agave, milk, salt, and vanilla. Blend until relatively smooth but don't overdo it or it will turn into cashew butter.

For the lemon cashew filling:

2 cups cashews

2 cups water

2 tablespoons agave nectar

¼ cup almond milk (or your favorite nondairy milk)

⅛ teaspoon salt

½ teaspoon pure vanilla extract

1 lemon

For everything else:

1 recipe Crepes (page 104)

1 recipe Whole Berry Sauce (page 202)

Powdered sugar for sprinkling

The mixture should be a thick and creamy consistency with just a bit of graininess.

Transfer to a mixing bowl. Use a microplane to finely grate the lemon zest in, about 2 teaspoons. Add juice from half of the lemon and mix well. Taste for lemon and add more of the juice if you like. Refrigerate until ready to use.

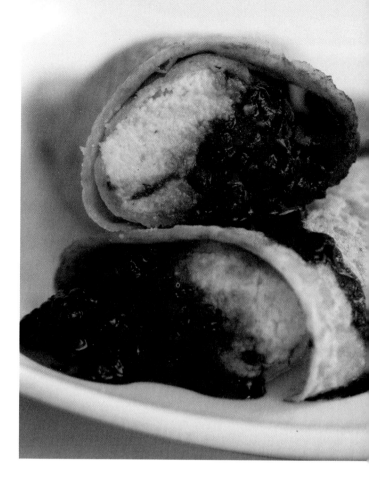

TO ASSEMBLE

For rolled crepes

On the lower third of the crepe, place about ¼ cup's worth of cashew filling in a log shape. Pour about ¼ cup of berry sauce over the filling and gently roll upwards. Repeat with remaining crepes and sprinkle with powdered sugar to serve.

For folded crepes

This isn't an exact science (it's kind of sloppy and imprecise, with berry sauce pouring out the edges), but it's still pretty and no one will complain. Place about ¼ cup of cashew filling on lower half of the crepe. Pour about ¼ cup of berry sauce over the filling. Fold the top half over and then fold in half so that the crepe is triangular. Repeat with remaining crepes and sprinkle with powdered sugar to serve.

The Sides

Potatoes, Sausages, and
a Stuffed Veggie or Two—
Everything You Need
to Make Brunch Complete

Roasted Potatoes

Serves 4

I don't want to get too dramatic here, but brunch is simply not worth living without potatoes. Roasted potatoes are a great choice for morning spuds because you can just shove them in the oven and not have to fuss. This recipe features my basic method—bite-size chunks, a little olive oil, salt and pepper, and super-high heat. There are endless flavor combinations you can try once you've got the method down, but I've listed a few of my favorites to start with.

2½ pounds Yukon Gold potatoes
2 tablespoons olive oil
½ teaspoon salt
Fresh black pepper, to taste

Preheat the oven to 425°F.

Line an 11 x 17-inch baking sheet with parchment paper. If you don't have parchment paper, spray the sheet with cooking spray or lightly grease with olive oil.

Slice potatoes in half lengthwise and then into about ¾-inch pieces. Place on baking sheet and drizzle with oil. Use your hands to coat the potatoes in the oil, then sprinkle them with salt.

Bake potatoes in the oven for 20 minutes. At this point, remove the tray from the oven and use a spatula to flip the potatoes. You don't have to be too precise about this—if some don't flip it's fine, just hope for the best.

Return potatoes to the oven and roast for 10 to 15 more minutes, until lightly browned outside and tender and creamy inside. Grind pepper over the potatoes to taste.

TIP I really like to use parchment paper on the baking sheet because it ensures that nothing sticks to the pan. And sometimes, if you're careful, you don't even need to clean the baking sheet afterwards. Is that too much information? Okay, well don't tell anyone I do that.

This recipe is for larger potatoes, but you can also whole roast baby potatoes or fingerlings that are on the smaller side. Use the same preparation and ingredients listed, only save yourself the trouble of cutting the potatoes and just roast them whole and unpeeled.

☼ VARIATIONS ☼

PAPRIKA ROSEMARY POTATOES

Once coated with oil and salt, sprinkle potatoes with **2½ teaspoons sweet paprika**, **½ teaspoon ground cumin**, and **2 teaspoons dried rosemary** crushed between your fingers. Toss to coat. No pepper is needed.

GARLIC ROASTED POTATOES

After the first 20 minutes of baking, flip the potatoes and bake for 7 more minutes. Coat **4 minced garlic cloves** with **1 teaspoon olive oil**. Sprinkle over potatoes and return to oven for 8 to 13 more minutes. Toss well before serving. You can use the garlic variation along with any other variation listed.

LEMON PEPPER ROASTED POTATOES

This one's easy. Omit the black pepper from the recipe and if your lemon pepper is salted, then omit the salt, too. After oiling the potatoes, sprinkle them with **1½ tablespoons lemon pepper**. Toss to coat.

CURRY ROASTED POTATOES

Another simple one. Omit black pepper from the recipe. After sprinkling potatoes with salt, sprinkle with **1 tablespoon curry powder** and **½ teaspoon ground cumin**. Toss to coat.

FRESH HERB ROASTED POTATOES

Adding the herbs at the end of the roasting process helps them keep their flavor. After the first 20 minutes of baking, flip the potatoes and bake for 7 more minutes. Remove from oven once more and sprinkle the potatoes with **1 tablespoon chopped fresh thyme**, **1 tablespoon chopped fresh rosemary**, and **1 tablespoon chopped fresh marjoram** (or any combination thereof). Toss to coat and bake for another 8 to 13 minutes. Toss before serving.

Individual Baked Hash Browns

Makes 12 muffin-size servings

Yeah, hash browns dripping with oil are great but sometimes you don't want a brunch you'll be paying for the rest of the day. These are baked and really simple; the real work is squeezing the water out of the potatoes. Once you've done that you'll have crisp-on-the-outside, tender-on-the-inside, pure potato bliss. Use Yukon Gold because then no peeling is required. If you sub with russets, you'll have to peel them.

3 pounds Yukon Gold potatoes, scrubbed

¼ cup vegetable oil (canola is good)

1 tablespoon cornstarch

1 teaspoon salt

½ teaspoon ground black pepper

Note: If you need the oven to be at 350°F because you're baking something else with these, that's fine. Just cook for 10 or so minutes longer.

Preheat the oven to 400°F. Liberally grease a muffin tin.

First, the potatoes need to be grated. And they really should be more grated than shredded, so if you are using a food processor, first cut them into ¾-inch chunks and then shred them with the shredding attachment (this method will yield a smaller cube more akin to grating). You can also grate them with a box grater.

Place the grated potatoes in cheesecloth or a large kitchen towel. Gather up the edges and wring the potatoes over the sink. Water should ooze out. It might take up to 3 minutes to drain out enough water and your hands may cramp, but soldier on! Squeeze the potatoes by the handful until very little moisture is left. Once they are well drained they are ready.

The rest of the recipe is easy. Place the drained potatoes in a large mixing bowl and add the remaining ingredients. Mix well. Divvy up the potatoes into the muffin tin, filling it all the way. Bake for 30 to 35 minutes, until the tops are golden brown.

Let hash browns cool for about 10 minutes. As soon as they are cool enough to handle (but still warm) use a paring knife to scrape around their edges and unstick them from the tin, then use a fork to coax them out.

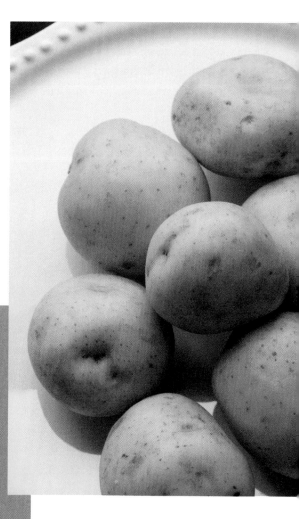

TIP Use Yukon Gold potatoes for this recipe because then no peeling is required. If you sub with russets, you'll have to peel them.

Potato Spinach Squares

Makes 16 pieces

These squares are almost like crustless knishes—each is a dense wedge of potatoes laced with spinach, oregano, and lemon. Because these taste great at room temperature, they're a perfect choice for a potluck. Puttanesca Scramble (page 29) makes a great main dish, even though these potatoes will vie for the spotlight.

In a large pot, cover the potatoes in water and bring them to a boil. Once boiling, lower the heat to simmer for about 20 minutes, or until potatoes are easily pierced with a fork. Drain and place potatoes in a large mixing bowl. Preheat the oven to 400°F.

Use a potato masher or a strong fork to mash the potatoes a bit. Add nutritional yeast and oil and continue to mash until creamy. Press the thawed spinach in a colander to remove some of the water. Combine with the potatoes. Add oregano, lemon juice, zest, salt, and several dashes of pepper. Mix in 1 cup of the breadcrumbs and thoroughly combine. Taste and adjust seasonings if necessary.

Lightly grease a 9 × 13-inch baking pan with cooking spray. Spread potatoes in evenly and sprinkle with ¼ cup breadcrumbs and a few pinches of paprika. Spray with cooking spray to moisten the breadcrumbs. Bake for 30 minutes. The dish is ready when the top is browned and the potatoes are pulling away from the sides of the pan. Let cool for at least 10 minutes before slicing into squares and serving, but a word to the wise: this dish tastes better the longer you let it cool. Sprinkle with fresh oregano to serve, if you like.

3 pounds yellow potatoes (like Yukon Gold), cut into ¾-inch chunks

¼ cup nutritional yeast

¼ cup olive oil

1 16-ounce package chopped frozen spinach, thawed

3 tablespoons chopped fresh oregano (or 1 tablespoon dried)

2 tablespoons fresh lemon juice (juice from 1 lemon)

Zest from 1 lemon

1½ teaspoons salt

Fresh black pepper

1¼ cups breadcrumbs, divided

A few pinches paprika

Additional fresh oregano for garnish (optional)

Diner Home Fries

Serves 4 to 6

This is how we do it in Brooklyn. Boiled and lightly fried potatoes with green peppers and onions. It's pretty bare bones, but no breakfast would be complete without them. Use your biggest pan (you don't want the pan to be crowded) so that everything cooks faster. If you know the night before that you'll be preparing these for breakfast, boil the potatoes in advance, drain them, and keep them covered in an airtight plastic container overnight. Bring them to room temperature before cooking to make things faster. I like to drizzle malt vinegar over them sometimes and get all Irish.

2 pounds Yukon Gold potatoes (about 4 to 6 potatoes), cut in half lengthwise, sliced ⅓ inch thick or so

3 tablespoons vegetable oil, divided

1 green pepper, seeded, cut into ¼-inch wide, inch-long pieces

1 medium onion, cut into ½-inch wide, inch-long pieces

¾ teaspoon salt

½ teaspoon ground black pepper

Place potatoes in a pot and cover with cold water. Cover the pot and bring to a boil. Once boiling, turn heat down just a bit (to medium high) and cook for about 15 more minutes, until potatoes are thoroughly cooked but still firm. Drain well.

Preheat a large, heavy-bottomed skillet over medium-high heat. Add 2 tablespoons oil and let the oil get hot. Add the potatoes and flip them around with a spatula to coat in oil. Let them cook undisturbed for about 5 to 7 minutes; they should be lightly browned. If not then bring the heat up a bit. Toss them and let cook for 10 more minutes, flipping occasionally to brown all sides. They won't all get browned and crispy; just do your best.

Add the peppers, onions, salt and pepper, and another tablespoon of oil and cook for 5 to 7 more minutes, stirring often, until onions and peppers are cooked.

Peruvian Home Fries

Serves 4 to 6

From the farmers' market to the supermarket, the sultry blue potato is coming out of hiding and staking its claim on produce shelves. Blue potatoes can sometimes be purple potatoes and vice versa, but don't worry about all that; if it looks even remotely like a black eye, you can call it a blue potato.

Here we take the traditional North American home fry and give it a Latin American spin. Colorful red onion and red bell peppers, aromatic coriander seeds, and a little heat from red pepper flakes make these Peruvian natives the perfect sidekick to Courico Tacos with Grilled Pineapple Salsa (page 73), an Omelet Rancheros (page 16), or any Latin-inspired spread.

2 pounds blue potatoes cut in ¾-inch pieces

3 tablespoons vegetable oil, divided

2 teaspoons coriander seeds, crushed

½ teaspoon red pepper flakes

1 red bell pepper, seeded, cut into ½-inch wide, inch-long pieces

1 medium red onion, cut into ½-inch wide, inch-long pieces

¾ teaspoon salt

Cilantro for garnish (optional)

Place potatoes in a pot and cover with cold water. Cover the pot and bring to a boil. Once boiling, turn heat down to simmer and cook for about 10 to 12 more minutes—they should be thoroughly cooked but still firm. Drain well.

Preheat a large, heavy-bottomed skillet over medium-high heat. Add 2 tablespoons oil and let the oil get hot. Add the coriander seeds, red pepper flakes, and potatoes. Flip them around with a spatula to coat in oil. Let them cook undisturbed for about 5 to 7 minutes; they should be lightly browned. If not then bring the heat up a bit. Toss them and let cook for 10 more minutes, flipping occasionally to brown all sides. They won't all get browned and crispy; just do your best.

Add the peppers, onions, and salt, plus another tablespoon of oil, and cook for 5 to 7 more minutes, stirring often, until onions and peppers are cooked. Garnish with fresh cilantro if you like.

Red Flannel Hash

Serves 6

I love the title "flannel hash"—it makes me think of forest men coming home to a hearty breakfast after a full day out in the woods logging the trees and destroying the planet. Beets and potatoes are diced up with some onion, sautéed on the stovetop, and then baked for a bit to get crispy. But you can eat them after the stovetop cooking if they are softened and you are pressed for time. I throw in a little liquid smoke at the end, but don't worry about it if you don't have any.

2 tablespoons olive oil

1½ pounds yellow potatoes, diced into ½-inch pieces (about 2 large)

1 medium-size beet, diced into ½-inch pieces

1 medium yellow onion, diced

½ teaspoon salt

Fresh black pepper

1 teaspoon liquid smoke (optional)

Preheat a large oven-safe skillet (cast iron, for instance) over medium heat. Cover the skillet and cook the potatoes and beets in the oil for about 15 minutes, stirring occasionally.

Add the onions and cook for another 15 minutes uncovered, stirring occasionally.

Preheat the oven to 350°F.

Add salt, pepper, and liquid smoke and stir to combine. Taste and adjust seasonings if you like. Place in the oven and cook for 10 to 20 more minutes, uncovered, or until potatoes and beets are very tender. I know 10 to 20 is a big window of time, but it varied a lot with our testers depending on the oven—check on your hash to make sure it doesn't burn.

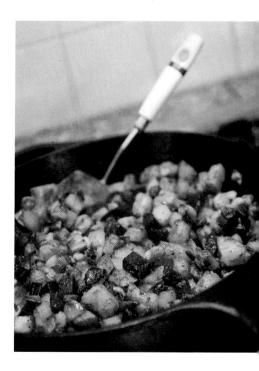

Coleslaw Potato Salad with Cumin Seeds

Serves 8

That's right, potato salad and coleslaw together at last. What took them so long? Everyone else could see it coming. This version is specifically for the Ethiopian Crepes (page 77); the toasty cumin seeds penetrate the dressing and add a deep, smoky flavor. Steaming the potatoes helps them keep their shape while staying smooth and creamy inside. It would also pair well with any Latin American dish.

Make ahead: Steam potatoes the evening before and refrigerate overnight. Toast cumin seeds the evening before and store in a plastic bag.

1 pound bite-size whole red potatoes (see note)

½ cup Vegenaise mayonnaise

2 tablespoons white vinegar

2 teaspoons sugar

4 cups coleslaw mix or shredded cabbage (see note)

Fresh black pepper

1 tablespoon cumin seeds, toasted

Salt, to taste

Chopped fresh mint for garnish (optional)

Steam potatoes for about 15 minutes or until tender. If you don't have a steamer, just simmer them in water for 15 minutes. Place in the fridge to cool completely.

Mix together the mayo, vinegar, and sugar. Add coleslaw and use tongs to mix well. Add the pepper and the cumin seeds and toss to coat. Add potatoes, toss again, and taste for salt. Refrigerate for at least 15 minutes to give the flavors a chance to marry. Garnish with chopped fresh mint if desired.

TIP Try to choose potatoes that are no bigger than a walnut. If small potatoes aren't available, just chop normal-size potatoes into roughly ¾-inch chunks.

Coleslaw mix is typically red and white cabbage plus shredded carrots. This combo looks really pretty, but if you can't find it then shredded cabbage of either color will work. You can also add a handful of shredded carrot for color.

To dry toast cumin seeds, preheat a small pan over medium heat. Add seeds and toast for about 3 minutes, stirring often, until seeds are fragrant and a few shades darker. Remove from heat immediately.

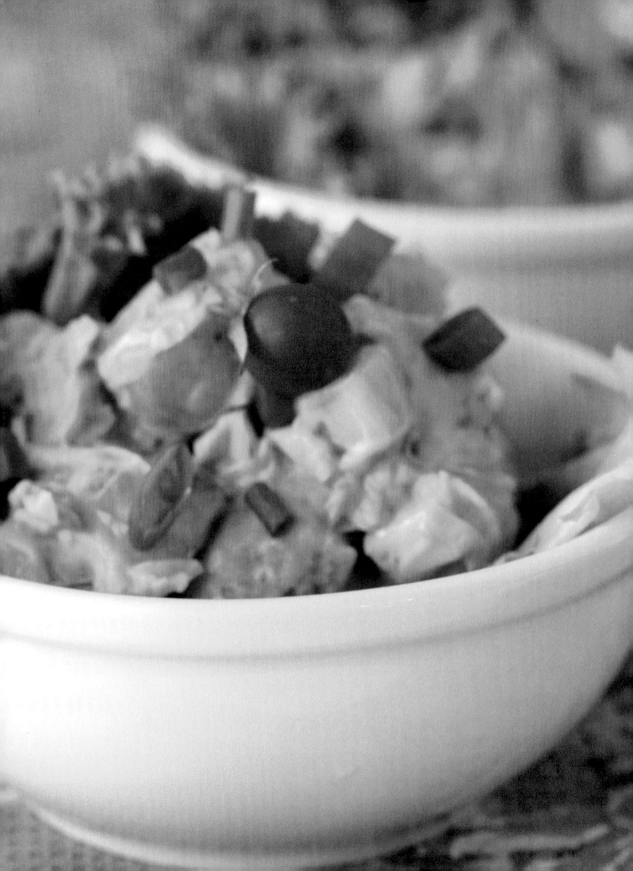

Creamy Avocado Potato Salad

Serves 6 to 8

Am I a genius or what? Come on, just say it! Potato salad with creamy guac instead of mayo? Seriously. The secret to the creaminess of this salad is a food processor. If you don't have one use a blender, but it's important to get the avocado as smooth as possible.

Note: Prepare this as close to serving time as possible. It can sit for a couple of hours, but anything longer and the avocado will brown.

2 pounds fingerling potatoes, cut into ¾-inch chunks

2 avocados

2 tablespoons lime juice, from a lime or two

½ teaspoon salt

¼ teaspoon ground cayenne (optional)

1 plum tomato, chopped

1 small red onion, diced small

1 smallish cucumber, diced very small

Put the potatoes in a pot and cover them with water. Cover the pot and bring the water to a boil. Lower the heat to a rolling boil and cook for 15 to 20 minutes, until potatoes are easily pierced with a fork. Drain and set aside to cool.

Once the potatoes have cooled, prepare the dressing. Split the avocados in half, remove the pits, and scoop the yumminess into the food processor. Add the lime juice and salt and puree until smooth, scraping down the sides with a spatula as needed. Once smooth and creamy, add the cayenne (if using), tomato, and onion. Pulse until they are incorporated but not completely blended. You should still be able to see the tomato and onion.

Put the potatoes and cucumbers in a large mixing bowl and mix them up. Add the avocado dressing and mix well. Taste for salt. Chill until ready to use.

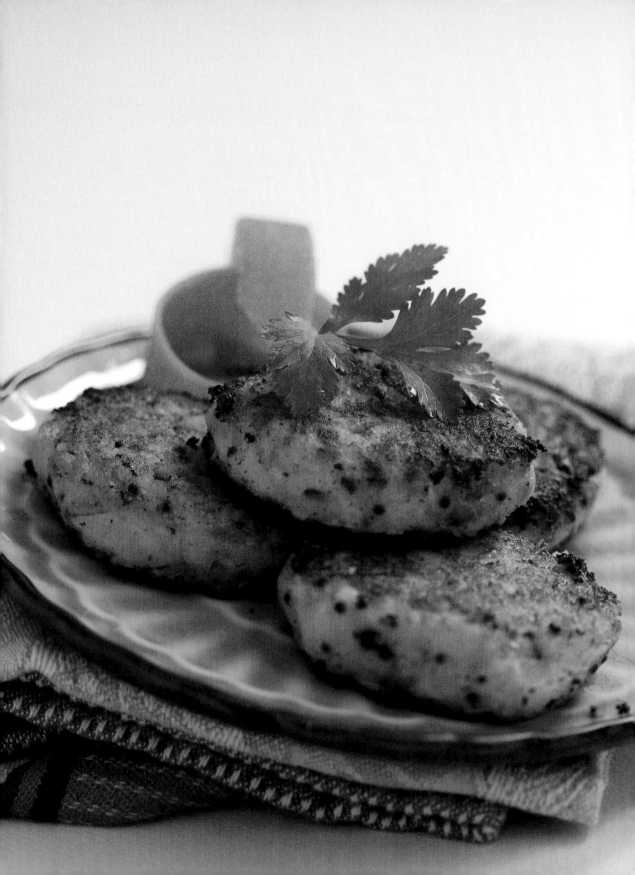

Samosa Mashed Potato Pancakes

Makes 30 pancakes

These are a really fun little treat for an Indian-inspired brunch. Samosa filling is formed into little cakes and panfried, giving you all the taste of a samosa and none of the hard work of dough making. They make a great finger food if you spike each with a toothpick, or a wonderful side to the Curried Cauliflower Frittata (page 38). Serve with your favorite chutney or try the Spiced Apple Cider Chutney (page 72). This recipe scales down or up perfectly, so if it's a brunch for four then you can halve this with no problem.

Make ahead: The potato mixture will need to chill at least one hour. You can prepare the entire mixture the night before so that it has ample time to cool. In the morning, just form into cakes, panfry, and serve.

What we'll be doing is making a mashed potato base and adding popped mustard seeds and sautéed veggies to that. So get a big pot for your potatoes and cover them in cold water. Bring to a boil. Once boiling, lower the heat to medium and simmer for 20 more minutes, or until potatoes are tender.

In the meantime, we'll pop the mustard seeds and cook the veggies. Preheat a large, heavy-bottomed skillet (preferably cast iron) over medium-high heat.

For the mashed potato base:

4 pounds Yukon Gold potatoes, peeled, cut into 1-inch chunks

¼ cup canola oil

¼ teaspoon turmeric

1 teaspoon salt, or to taste

For everything else:

2 tablespoons canola oil

2 teaspoons yellow mustard seeds

1 medium onion, finely chopped

1 cup carrot, diced small

4 garlic cloves, minced

1-inch square piece of fresh ginger, peeled and minced

2 teaspoons ground cumin

½ teaspoon red pepper flakes

¾ cup frozen peas

¼ cup all-purpose flour

Extra canola oil for panfrying

Chopped fresh cilantro for garnish (optional)

(Have a lid handy.) Add the 2 tablespoons canola oil. Wait about 15 seconds for oil to heat up, then spoon in the mustard seeds. Cover with the lid and let the seeds pop for about a minute. If they aren't popping, the heat isn't high enough, so turn it up. Once the popping settles down, add the onion and carrot. Sauté for about 10 minutes until the onion is browned and the carrot is slightly softened. Add the garlic, ginger, cumin, and red pepper flakes. Cook for another 5 minutes, mixing frequently. Sprinkle in some water if the vegetables appear dry. Once done, cover until ready to use.

Now return to the potatoes. Once they are tender, drain and return to the pot. Mash well. Add the canola oil, turmeric, and salt and mash until relatively smooth. Stir in the onion mixture and the frozen peas (they will thaw when you mix them in). Add the flour and mix well (use your hands to mix at this point; it's just easier). Taste for salt.

The mixture needs to cool completely before proceeding or it will fall apart, so it's a good idea to make these the night before. Otherwise, let them sit in the fridge for at least an hour and give them a mix every now and again to hasten cooling.

Once cooled, roll handfuls of potato mixture into golf ball–size balls. If you're having problems with the mixture being too moist and difficult to roll, then add a little extra flour by the tablespoonful. Flatten the balls out a bit and roll the sides in your palms into roughly 1¾-inch-wide tire shapes to form cakes.

Preheat a large, heavy-bottomed skillet over medium heat. Add a thin layer of oil, just enough to coat the bottom of the pan, and cook cakes for about 3 to 4 minutes on each side, until golden brown and heated through. Do this in several batches to avoid crowding the pan. Transfer to absorbent paper (paper towels or a paper bag) and cover with a plate or some tinfoil to keep warm while you make the others.

When they're all done, sprinkle with chopped cilantro if you like, and serve.

TIP To make these gluten-free and add a little flavor, use chickpea flour instead of all-purpose flour to bind.

Jalapeño Garlic Grits

Serves 4 to 6

Yeah, good old-fashioned grits. The kind enjoyed at truck stops across the nation. And we vegans know it, too, since during our road trips to and from Portland they are often the only vegan item on the menu. These are done up with lots of garlic and some jalapeño for a little kick to your comfort food. Serve in a big old bowl and let guests ladle it out mess hall–style. I ask that you follow the directions on the package to cook the grits, since they do vary from brand to brand.

In a saucepot over medium heat, sauté garlic and jalapeños in oil for about 3 minutes, until garlic is lightly browned. Mix in the grits, along with salt and nutritional yeast (if using). Taste for salt. Keep covered until ready to serve and make sure to serve nice and hot.

1 cup dry grits, cooked according to package directions

2 tablespoons vegetable oil

6 garlic cloves, minced

3 jalapeños, seeded and thinly sliced

1 teaspoon salt

2 tablespoons nutritional yeast (optional)

TIP For extra flavor, use vegetable broth to cook your grits instead of plain old water.

The Nitty Gritty

Although both Italian polenta and American grits are made from corn and both are called grits, there are some differences. Cornmeal for polenta is just ground-up dried corn, no big deal. Grits, though prepared the same way, are made from hominy, which is corn kernels soaked in an alkaline solution (usually baking soda, wood ash, or lime-water) until they swell up and the shell pops off. The swollen kernels are then dried and ground into meal. This process gives grits their well-known fluffy demeanor.

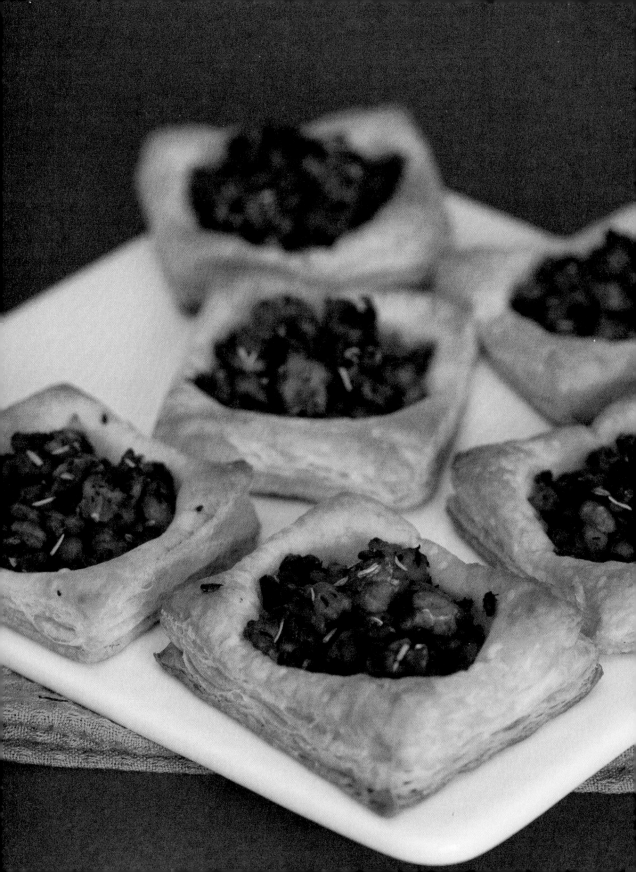

Tempeh Sausage Pastry Puffs

Makes 18 pastries

Cute little squares that are both flaky and hearty. They'd make a good main event with some greens and gravy, or a fun brunch starter if you have a bunch of people over. The fennel and herb tempeh is reminiscent of the winter holidays, making these the perfect choice for a Thanksgiving brunch. I have traditionally been against puff pastry in recipes, but let's be honest, none of us can make anything as light, flaky, and fun all by ourselves. If serving as a main, then I would say two each is the way to go.

Note: Don't forget to thaw your pastry before starting this recipe. I thaw it overnight in the fridge, but you can also thaw for 30 minutes on your countertop.

Whisk the marinade ingredients together in a small mixing bowl. Add the tempeh and let marinate for an hour.

When the hour is almost up, preheat a large pan over medium heat. Sauté the red bell pepper and onion in the oil for 7 to 10 minutes, until the onion is translucent. Add garlic and spices and sauté another 3 minutes. Drain the marinated tempeh and add it to the pan. Turn the heat up to medium high and cook for about 15 minutes, stirring often.

8 ounces tempeh, crumbled

1 package puff pastry (Pepperidge Farm brand is vegan), thawed

For the marinade:

1 cup vegetable broth

3 tablespoons soy sauce

2 tablespoons lemon juice

For everything else:

2 tablespoons olive oil

1 red bell pepper, finely chopped

1 small onion, finely chopped

3 garlic cloves, minced

2 teaspoons fennel seeds, chopped

2 teaspoons dried thyme

2 teaspoons dried rosemary

½ teaspoon red pepper flakes

Salt, to taste

Olive oil for brushing the pastry

In the meantime, preheat the oven to 400°F and start preparing your puff pastries. Pour a little olive oil into a cup and brush a large baking sheet with olive oil. Cut each pastry sheet into nine squares and set them on the baking sheet at least an inch apart. Brush the tops of the pastries with olive oil. When the tempeh is ready, taste for salt and remove from heat. Top each pastry right in the middle with a heaping tablespoon of tempeh.

Bake for 18 to 20 minutes, until the pastries are nice and puffed. Serve ASAP.

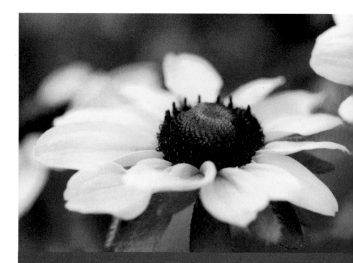

TIP I think lemon pepper is one of those spices whose flavor is drastically different depending on what brand you buy, and the cheapo brands never seem as flavorful as the higher-end ones and can even taste downright dusty. Yet the classier brands aren't even that much more expensive. Look for the kind in a glass, not plastic, jar or order from Penzeys Spices, my favorite brand.

Lemon Pepper Tofu

Serves 2 as a main, 4 as a side

This recipe is so ridiculously easy that I feel almost silly putting it in a book. It's a really fast way to have some really flavorful tofu to go along with your brunch—stuffed into burritos, beside your pancakes, in a sammich, over a salad, topped off on the Polenta Rancheros (page 51), and on and on. Since brunch can be really time consuming, this tofu is a lifesaver that can be popped into the oven and left to its own devices. You don't even need to press the tofu. I'm giving you the amounts here, but once you make it you can really just eyeball the ingredients; no need to measure.

1 pound extra-firm tofu, sliced into 8 pieces widthwise

2 teaspoons olive oil

1 teaspoon Bragg Liquid Aminos (or soy sauce, if you like)

2 garlic cloves

2 tablespoons lemon pepper (with salt)

Preheat the oven to 350°F. Spray a baking sheet with cooking spray or lightly coat with oil. Poke each slice of tofu with a fork 3 to 4 times to let the flavors seep in.

Drizzle the olive oil and liquid aminos on a plate. Use a microplane to grate the garlic into the mix. If you don't have a microplane, then just mince the garlic to as close to a paste as you can. Dredge each slice of tofu and lay them out on the plate. Sprinkle one tablespoon of the lemon pepper over the tofu and give it a quick rub into the tofu. Flip the slices and sprinkle on the second tablespoon. Now rub each slice really well—don't forget about the edges of the tofu, get those, too. I usually spend about 15 seconds on each slice.

Place tofu in a single layer on the baking sheet. Bake for 20 minutes on one side, flip over, and bake another 10 minutes. Remove from oven and cover with tinfoil until ready to serve.

Chesapeake Tempeh Cakes

Makes 10 cakes

I love the succulent little pieces of tempeh you get when biting into this crisp, flavorful cake. Crab cakes are the inspiration here, although I've never actually had one. I used to spend lots of time in Baltimore, which is famous for its crabs, and back then pollution in the Chesapeake Bay was a big issue. I think it's doing much better now and these cakes are a tribute to it.

Make ahead: Make the entire mixture and the remoulade the night before. In the morning, form into cakes and panfry.

First we're going to steam the tempeh to get the bitterness out and also to give it some flavor with the soy sauce. Crumble the tempeh into a saucepan in little bits. Add the water, soy sauce, oil, and bay leaf. The tempeh won't be fully submerged, but that's fine. Cover and bring to a boil. Once boiling, let boil for 12 to 15 minutes, until most of the water has evaporated. Stir once during boiling.

Transfer contents to a mixing bowl, remove the bay leaf, and mash with a fork. Let cool for about 15 minutes, stirring occasionally to hasten the cooling process. Make sure the tempeh is barely warm before you proceed, or the cakes may fall apart when you cook them. Add the Vegenaise, mustard, hot sauce, vinegar,

For the cakes:

8 ounces tempeh (use the nori tempeh if you can find it, but plain soy tempeh is fine, too)

1 cup water

1 tablespoon soy sauce

1 tablespoon olive oil

1 bay leaf

3 tablespoons Vegenaise

1 tablespoon whole-grain mustard (stone-ground Dijon works, too)

1 tablespoon hot sauce

1 tablespoon red wine vinegar

¼ cup very finely chopped red bell pepper

¾ teaspoon ground ginger

½ teaspoon dried oregano

½ teaspoon salt

Fresh black pepper

1½ cups panko breadcrumbs, plus extra for dredging

1 finely chopped nori sheet or 1 tablespoon kelp granules (optional, if you like a little fishiness)

Oil for panfrying

2 tablespoons Vegenaise

1 tablespoon whole-grain
    mustard (stone-ground Dijon
    works, too)

1 tablespoon hot sauce

2 teaspoons capers (try not to get
    too much brine)

For serving:

Lemon wedges

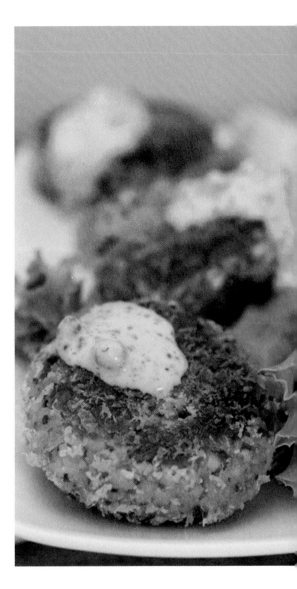

bell pepper, ginger, oregano, salt, and pepper and mix well. Add the breadcrumbs and nori, if using, and use your hands to incorporate.

Once you are ready to form the cakes, preheat a thin layer of oil in a heavy-bottomed, nonstick skillet (cast iron is great) over medium heat. Pour a few tablespoons of panko into a bowl. Scoop a little less than ¼ cup batter into your hands and form into a ball. Flatten between your palms and then roll the sides gently to smooth them. You should have ten 2½- to 3-inch patties. Press them into the panko to lightly coat. They don't need to be thoroughly covered, just a little bit for some texture.

Fry a batch of five cakes for 4 minutes on one side and flip when dark golden brown. Fry for 2 minutes on the other side and transfer to a paper towel or paper bag to drain. Do your second batch and in the meantime make your remoulade by mixing all the ingredients together in a bowl.

Serve with lemon wedges.

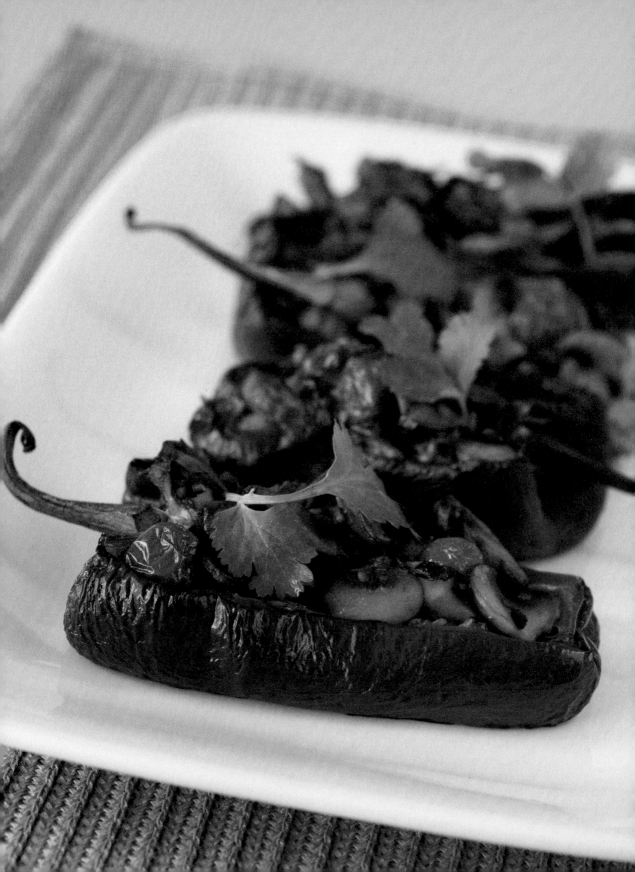

Poblanos Stuffed with Coriander Seeds and Mushrooms

Serves 4

Poblanos roast differently than regular green peppers. They're more tender and have a little kick, plus their ballet slipper shape is just a little more fun. Cremini mushrooms provide a juicy filling and a handful of shiitakes lend some meatiness. Serve with Peruvian Home Fries (page 118), Fried Plantains (page 151), and Guacamole (page 221).

Make ahead: Prepare the mushrooms the night before. Refrigerate in a covered container overnight.

Preheat a large, heavy-bottomed skillet over medium-low heat. Sauté the garlic, peppers, and coriander seeds in oil for about 5 minutes to soften the seeds. Stir frequently to avoid burning the garlic. Turn the heat up to medium, add the mushrooms, oregano, salt, and pepper, and sauté for about 7 minutes, until mushrooms are softened.

Preheat the oven to 350°F. Lightly grease a rimmed baking sheet.

While the mushrooms are cooking, prepare the poblanos. Slice them in half lengthwise, leaving the stem

2 tablespoons olive oil

6 garlic cloves, minced

2 Serrano peppers, thinly sliced (remove seeds if you want less heat)

1 tablespoon coriander seeds, crushed

1 pound cremini mushrooms, sliced

¼ pound shiitake mushrooms, sliced

2 teaspoons dried oregano

¼ teaspoon salt, plus more to taste

Several dashes fresh black pepper

1 cup cherry tomatoes, sliced in half

1 tablespoon fresh lime juice

4 poblano peppers

Fresh cilantro for garnish (optional)

intact. Remove the seeds and use a paring knife to remove as much of the membrane as you can.

Now, return to the mushrooms. Once softened, add the cherry tomatoes and sauté for 5 minutes more. Add the lime juice and taste for salt. Spoon the mushroom mixture into the poblanos, nudging it into the crevices. Place the peppers on a baking sheet. If a pepper is tilting over to one side, stick a tooth-pick through the side to give it "legs" for balance.

Bake for 30 to 35 minutes. When ready, the peppers should appear darker and crinkly. Top with chopped fresh cilantro if desired, and serve that baby up.

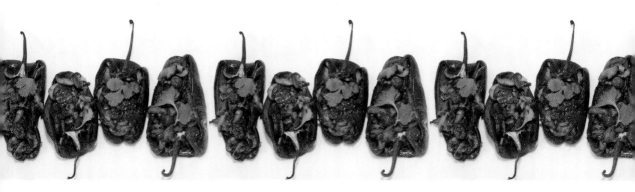

Sausages

Cookbook author (and friend!) Julie Hasson came up with the steaming method used in these sausage recipes, which offer several flavor variations that all share the same preparation instructions. It really is quite brilliant and much more economical than store-bought vegan sausages. I love that Julie shared the technique with the world. People are often too secretive about their discoveries, but the more improvements we can make to vegan cuisine the better. So if you see something, say something!

Cherry Sage Sausages

Makes 4 big sausages

Adding dried fruit to a sausage just seems so, I don't know, jubilant! These sausages will put a smile on all of your guests, even the ones who insist they aren't morning people and even if you have chosen "gothic" as your background music.

Before mixing your ingredients, get your steaming apparatus ready and bring water to a full boil. The rest of the recipe comes together very quickly.

Have ready four sheets of tinfoil. In a large bowl, mash the beans until no whole ones are left. Throw all the other ingredients together in the order listed and mix with a fork. Divide dough into four even parts (an easy way to do this: split the dough in half and then into quarters). Place one part of dough into tinfoil and mold into about a 5-inch log. Wrap dough in tinfoil, like a Tootsie Roll. Don't worry too much about shaping it; it will snap into shape while it's steaming because this recipe is awesome.

Place wrapped sausages in steamer and steam for 40 minutes. That's it! You can unwrap and enjoy immediately or refrigerate until ready to use. I like them sliced and sautéed in olive oil for a few minutes, or grilled whole and then sliced.

½ cup navy beans, rinsed and drained

1 cup vegetable broth

1 tablespoon olive oil

2 tablespoons soy sauce

1 teaspoon liquid smoke

2 garlic cloves, grated (with a microplane, or very finely minced)

1¼ cups vital wheat gluten

¼ cup nutritional yeast

1 tablespoon plus 1 teaspoon dry rubbed sage (*not* powdered)

½ teaspoon ground ginger

¼ teaspoon ground allspice

⅛ teaspoon ground cloves

Fresh black pepper

½ cup finely chopped dried cherries

Chorizo Sausages

Makes 4 big sausages

spicy sausage with just a little tomato kick. This sausage is a great way to add a little Spanish flair to your brunch buffet.

Follow same instructions as for Cherry Sage Sausages (page 138).

½ cup cooked pinto beans, rinsed and drained

1 cup vegetable broth

1 tablespoon olive oil

2 tablespoons soy sauce

2 tablespoons tomato paste

2 teaspoons lemon zest

2 garlic cloves, grated (with a microplane, or very finely minced)

1¼ cups vital wheat gluten

¼ cup nutritional yeast

1 tablespoon smoked paprika

1 teaspoon crushed red pepper flakes

1 tablespoon dry rubbed sage (*not* powdered)

1 teaspoon dried oregano

¼ teaspoon cayenne (optional; don't use if you don't like heat)

Italian Feast Sausages

Makes 4 big sausages

When I was a kid my family would make our way across Brooklyn to foreign lands (like Bensonhurst) to go to "The Feast." It was basically a street fair, with the usual suspects: merry-go-rounds, dunking booths, haunted houses, and, oh yes, about a million food vendors serving delicious greasy foods that just might kill you. These sausages are a nod to the ones that they would serve at The Feast, only kinder and healthier.

If you don't have a steamer you can use a colander in a big pot. But a steamer is the kind of thing that's sold for pennies in any thrift shop, so try to procure one toot sweet!

Follow same instructions as for Cherry Sage Sausages (page 138).

- ½ cup cooked navy beans, rinsed and drained
- 1 cup vegetable broth
- 1 tablespoon olive oil
- 2 tablespoons soy sauce
- 2 garlic cloves, grated (with a microplane, or very finely minced)
- 1¼ cups vital wheat gluten
- ¼ cup nutritional yeast
- 2 teaspoons fennel seeds, crushed
- 1 teaspoon red pepper flakes
- 1 teaspoon sweet paprika
- 1 teaspoon dried oregano
- Several dashes fresh black pepper

Tempeh Bacon Revamped

Serves 6 to 8 as a side

No brunch is complete without a few slabs of smoky tempeh. This recipe is not completely unlike the tempeh bacon in *Vegan with a Vengeance*, but it has more basic ingredients. I also cut the tempeh widthwise into slightly thicker pieces than the *VWAV* ones because people seemed to have a hard time accomplishing the long thin slices.

In a wide shallow bowl, mix together all the marinade ingredients. Add the tempeh slices and marinate them for about an hour.

Preheat a large, heavy-bottomed pan over medium heat. Panfry the tempeh in oil for about 7 minutes, flipping occasionally and adding more marinade as you flip. That's it!

For the marinade:

3 tablespoons soy sauce

1 tablespoon liquid smoke

1 tablespoon pure maple syrup

1 tablespoon apple cider vinegar

1 tablespoon olive oil

1 tablespoon tomato paste

¾ cup vegetable broth

2 garlic cloves, crushed

To cook:

8 to 12 ounces tempeh, cut widthwise into ¼-inch slices

1 tablespoon olive oil

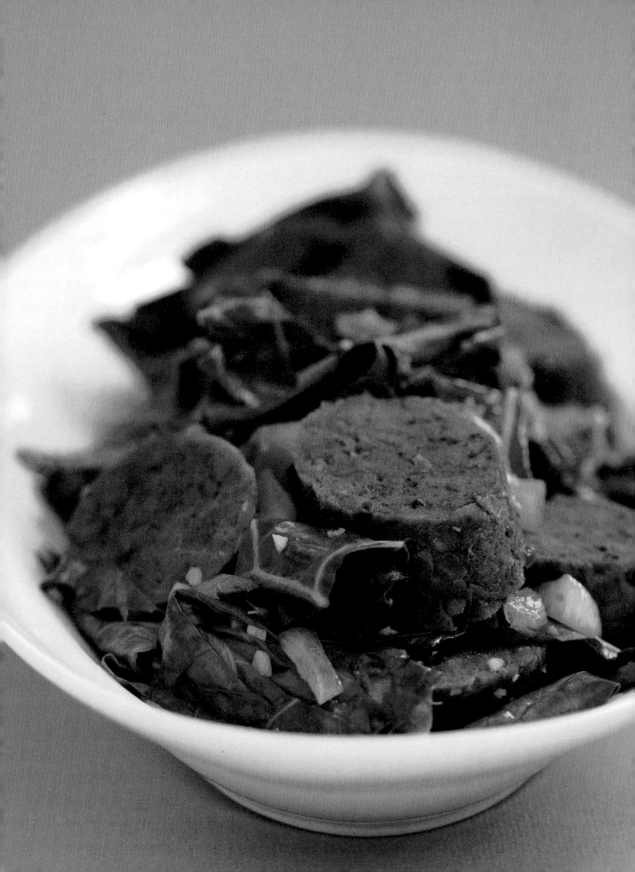

Sautéed Collards and Sausages

Serves 4

This is a succulent and Southern-inspired side to scrambled tofu and potatoes but would also be a wonderful main dish over soft polenta and with some biscuits and gravy. I use homemade Sausages (page 137–140), but you can use whatever vegan sausages you like. You can even cheat and use store-bought ones since I can't stop you.

Preheat a large pan over medium heat. Sauté the garlic and shallots in oil for about 3 minutes. Add the sausages and red pepper flakes and sauté for another 5 minutes or so, until sausages are lightly browned. It's okay if they break up a bit; in fact, it's good if they do.

Add collards, broth, and soy sauce and use tongs to stir. Cover the pan to get the collards to cook faster and cook for about 5 minutes, stirring occasionally. Once they've cooked down, remove the lid, turn the heat up, and use tongs to stir the collards and sausage around for about 3 minutes. The liquid should evaporate significantly.

Serve with slices of lemon.

2 tablespoons olive oil

6 garlic cloves, minced

2 shallots, finely chopped (about ¼ cup)

2 homemade sausages, chopped (pages 137–140)

Generous pinch red pepper flakes

1 bunch collards, chopped, rough stems removed

¼ cup veggie broth

1 tablespoon soy sauce

Lemon slices to serve

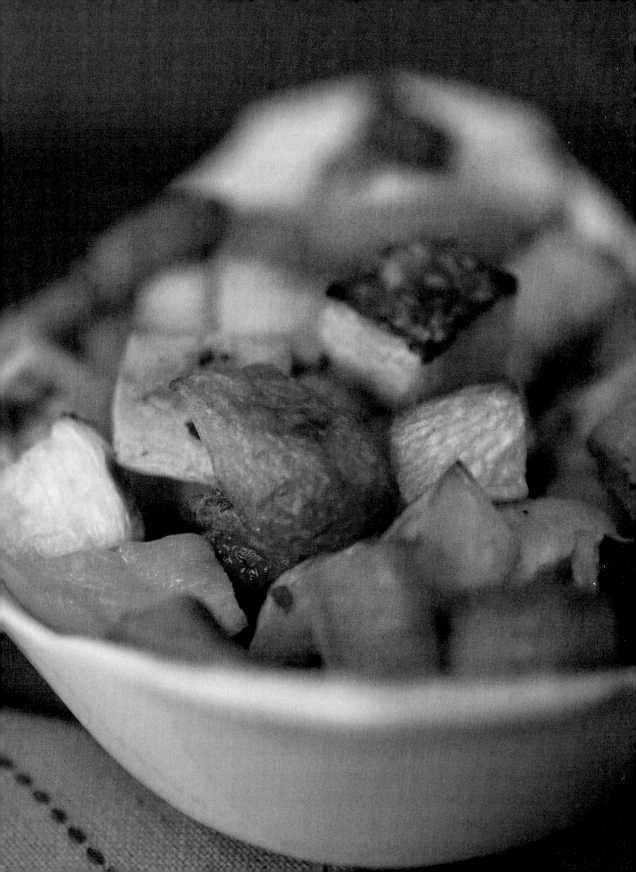

Roasted Root Vegetables

Serves 4 to 6

There's a sultry and exotic quality to these vegetables. They're cold-weather food to be sure, warming you from inside out and making you want to fall backwards into a huge pile of leaves and spend the day there. Sometimes I serve them simply—just pure roasted goodness with a little olive oil and salt. Other times I feel like dressing them up a bit with ginger and maple syrup. I give both options here. You can certainly double this recipe, or use whichever roots you like best.

Preheat the oven to 425°F. Line a large rimmed baking sheet with parchment paper.

Combine vegetables on the baking sheet, drizzle with olive oil and salt, then toss to coat. Use your hands to make sure you get everything.

Place in oven and bake for 30 minutes. Flip veggies with a spatula (you don't have to be too precise about it) and bake for about another 20 minutes or until soft and browned. The beets will take longest to cook, so give those a poke to make sure they're ready. Serve warm.

½ pound golden beets, peeled and cut into ¾-inch pieces

½ pound parsnips, peeled and cut into ¾-inch pieces

½ pound carrots, peeled and cut into ¾-inch pieces

½ pound rutabaga or turnip, peeled and cut into ¾-inch pieces

2 tablespoons olive oil

¾ teaspoon salt

For ginger maple roasted root vegetables add:

¼ cup pure maple syrup

2 tablespoons minced fresh ginger

Simple Stuffed Artichokes with Ginger and Chervil

Serves 4 to 6

Because trimming and prepping artichokes can be kind of a chore, it's nice to have a stuffing that isn't too fussy. But it does have a secret ingredient to shake things up a bit—ginger. That and garlic make this an aromatic, gingery stuffing, which also offers the delicate, lemony taste of chervil and the not-so-delicate, lemony taste of ... lemon. I like to just eat these artichokes with my hands, but have a fork nearby to scoop up any fallen stuffing. Never leave a man behind.

Note: If you've never stuffed an artichoke before, I'm going to direct you to a video so that you will not be intimidated. And it's kind of hard to explain anyway, so trust me, watch the video: http://allrecipes.com/HowTo/How-to-Cook-an-Artichoke-Video/Detail.aspx

2 cups breadcrumbs

1 tablespoon minced ginger

3 garlic cloves, minced

½ teaspoon salt

Fresh black pepper

2 tablespoons lemon juice

¼ cup olive oil

¼ cup chopped fresh chervil, plus extra for garnishing

4 big artichokes, or 6 smaller ones

First, get your vegetable steamer ready. Fill it with water and bring to a boil.

Next, prepare the artichoke stuffing. Just mix all the ingredients (except for the artichokes) together. That's it! Save the lemon that you juiced; you're gonna rub it on the artichokes.

Now, prep those artichokes. Slice about an inch and a half of the tops off and discard so that you can get to the "choke." (watch the video). Use a spoon (a grapefruit spoon works really well!) to scoop out the center; you should see some hairy stuff at the bottom of it—discard all of that. Cut about an inch off all remaining leaf tips with kitchen shears or scissors. After prepping each one, rub a little lemon juice on to prevent discoloring. But it's gonna discolor a little bit anyway, so don't sweat it too much.

Slice off the bottoms of the chokes, as little as possible, just so that they will stand up when you steam them. Gently spread the leaves of the artichokes apart and stuff that stuffing in there as much as you can.

Place stuffed artichokes in the steamer and cover. Small ones take about half an hour, large ones take about 50 minutes.

When they're done, garnish with chervil and dig in as fast as you can. You can squeeze more lemon juice over them if you wish.

Roasted Butternut Squash

Serves 4 to 6

1 medium-size butternut squash

2 tablespoons olive oil

½ teaspoon salt

Roasted butternut squash is like a big fluffy blanket on a wet autumn day. There's certainly nothing wrong with just splitting the squash, seeding it, and popping it in the oven. But when I've got the time I really love to peel and cube it; this way the outside is crisp and toasty and the inside is creamy and sweet. I also love to serve this in place of home fries. It tastes especially great alongside Basic Scrambled Tempeh (page 24).

Preheat the oven to 375°F. Peel the squash, then cut the round part from the long part. Cut the round part in half and scoop out the seeds. Slice everything into ½-inch to ¾-inch pieces.

Line a large baking sheet with parchment paper. Spread the squash out in a single layer and drizzle with olive oil. The single layer is important because if the baking sheet is overcrowded the squash won't brown, it'll steam and just get mushy. Sprinkle with salt and use your hands to coat everything.

Pop in the oven for about 45 minutes, flipping every 15 minutes or so. The squash is done when lightly browned on the outside and tender inside.

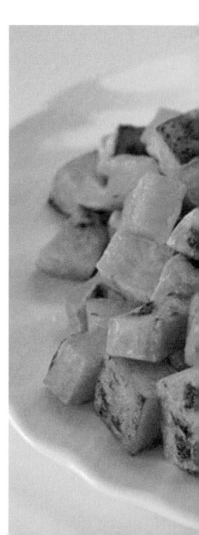

Roasted Portobellos

Serves 4 as a side

There's hardly ever a savory brunch dish that wouldn't benefit from a nice juicy portobello mushroom sliced on top. Serve over scrambled tofu or tempeh, or in an omelet, or with biscuits and gravy. Or just about anywhere.

2 large or 4 small portobello caps

For the marinade:

½ cup cooking wine

1 tablespoon olive oil

2 tablespoons soy sauce

2 tablespoons balsamic vinegar

2 garlic cloves, minced

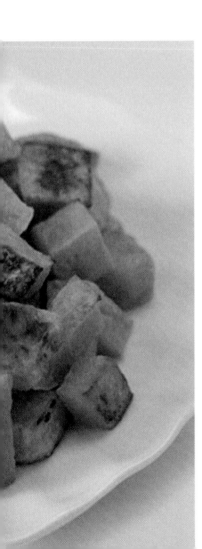

Combine all ingredients for the marinade in a glass pie plate or small casserole. Place the mushrooms upside down in the marinade and spoon a lot of the marinade into the cap so that there is a small pool. Preheat the oven to 400°F and marinate for about 20 minutes.

Cover with tinfoil and cook for ½ hour. Remove the tinfoil, use tongs to flip the caps over, and cook uncovered for another 10 minutes. Let it cool a bit and then slice very thinly on a bias to make nice meaty slivers.

Smoky Shiitakes

Serves 4

This is ideal brunch food: super-simple ingredients, minimal prep, quick cooking, and strong salty smoky flavor. The recipe doubles well, too. It's perfect over the Fennel Breakfast Risotto (page 48) or just as a smoky, salty side to your scrambled tofu or tempeh.

1 tablespoon canola oil (any vegetable oil will do)

8 ounces shiitake mushrooms, stems trimmed, sliced in half (about 3 cups)

1 tablespoon soy sauce

½ teaspoon liquid smoke

Preheat a heavy-bottomed skillet over medium-high heat. Add the oil and sauté the mushrooms for about 7 minutes, until they are soft. Add the soy sauce and liquid smoke and stir constantly until the soy sauce is absorbed (about 1 minute).

Fried Plantains

Serves 4 as a side

always crave a little sweetness with my brunches, even if I'm tucking into something savory. Fried plantains are a perfect option, with their crisp, caramelized exterior and sweet, pleasantly mushy interior. Choose plantains that are just beginning to blacken, so that they are sweet but still firm. These are delicious with Polenta Rancheros (page 51) or Courico Tacos with Grilled Pineapple Salsa (page 76), but also irresistible paired with Basic Scrambled Tofu (page 19) or Basic Scrambled Tempeh (page 24).

Slice the plantains on a bias into ½-inch slices. Preheat a heavy-bottomed skillet over medium-high heat. Add oil to the skillet until it's ¼ inch deep. When the oil is hot, add half the plantains or so; just don't overcrowd the pan.

Fry plantains about a minute, then flip; fry for about a minute longer, then flip again. This time press the plantains down into the skillet, being careful not to burn yourself with sputtering oil. They should be pressed down until they're about half as thick. Fry for 45 seconds or so and then flip yet again, fry for another 45 seconds, then transfer to a paper bag or paper towels to drain. Repeat with the remaining plantains. Sprinkle with salt, if you like. Serve ASAP.

2 plantains

Vegetable oil for shallow frying

Salt, to taste

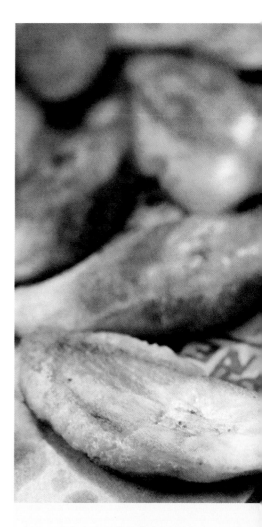

The Bread Basket

Scrumptiousness from the Oven,
from Muffins to Bagels

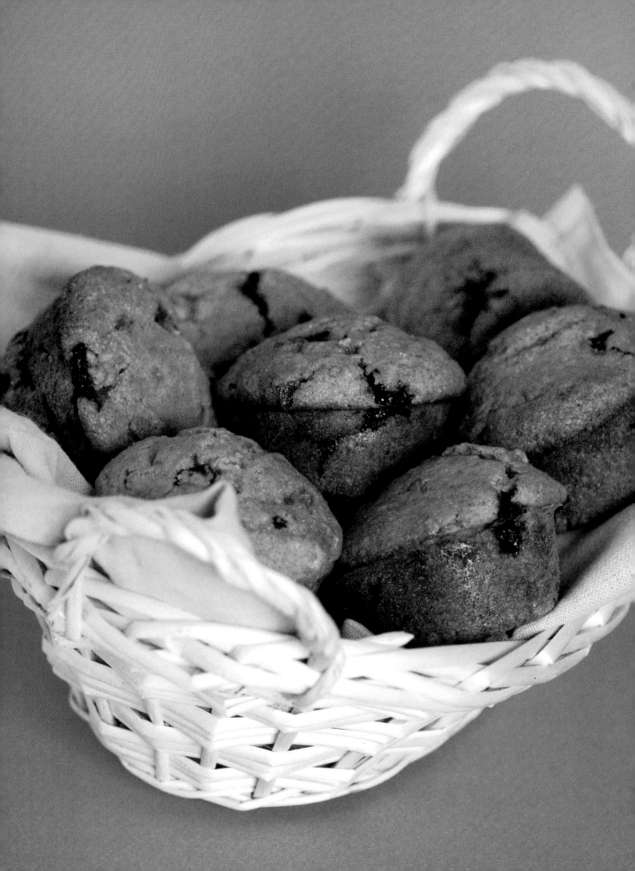

Blueberry Ginger Spelt Muffins

Makes 12 muffins

Spicy ginger and tart sweet blueberries are a perfect complement to each other. The ginger in these isn't a strong in-your-face wintry gingerbread sort of deal, it's just kind of like, "Hi, I'm ginger. Welcome to spring."

Preheat the oven to 375°F. Lightly grease a muffin tin.

In a large mixing bowl, stir together the flour, sugar, baking powder, salt, and spices. Make a well in the center and add the yogurt, milk, canola oil, and vanilla. Stir to combine. Fold in the ginger and the blueberries.

Scoop the batter into the muffin tin; it should almost fill the entire tin. Bake for 28 to 32 minutes, or until a toothpick or butter knife inserted through the center of the muffin comes out clean. Let cool for a few minutes in the tin before transferring the muffins to a cooling rack to cool completely.

2½ cups spelt flour (see spelt tip page 171)

½ cup sugar

1 tablespoon baking powder

½ teaspoon salt

2 teaspoons ground ginger

¼ teaspoon ground allspice

¼ teaspoon ground cinnamon

½ cup vanilla soy yogurt (a 6-ounce container)

1 cup almond milk (or your favorite nondairy milk)

⅓ cup canola oil

1 teaspoon pure vanilla extract

½ cup finely chopped crystallized ginger

1¼ cups blueberries

TIP Never buy the glass jars of crystallized ginger that are usually displayed with the spices; they are a total rip-off! Buy it in bulk or in the candy aisle.

Finding Your Thrills on (Frozen) Blueberry Hill

It's the middle of winter but you still want your blueberries! And rightfully so. That's where frozen blueberries come in. Often frozen berries taste even better than the off-season fresh variety because they were bagged and frozen at the height of their ripeness. There are just a few things to keep in mind while working with the little guys.

I don't mind a little bit of purple streaking in a blueberry muffin, that just adds to the fun. But to keep your muffins from becoming a mottled mess, keep the berries in the freezer until the last moment, not allowing them to thaw at all. This way the juices will be kept inside the berries, minimizing "bleeding" into the batter.

Don't use that bag of blueberries that's been sitting in the freezer since you were knee-high to a pair of legwarmers. Save that for the next time you have a sprained ankle or some other tragic injury that requires an ice pack. Buy a fresh bag that hasn't become freezer-burned or worse, a solid block of ice.

You don't have to be Bill Nye the Science Guy to figure out that adding frozen ingredients will lower the temperature of your muffin batter, thus necessitating a longer baking time. It usually takes only 3 to 5 minutes extra, but the toothpick test oughta take care of any doubts you might have as to whether or not those babies are done.

Many supermarkets have started carrying what they call "wild blueberries." I'm not sure about the wildness claim, but these berries are smaller and disperse more evenly in batter, so pick them up if you find them.

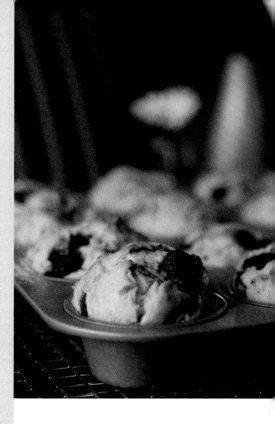

Timely Tips for Momentous Muffins

Use an ice cream scooper with a release trigger to pour batter into the muffin tins. This cuts down on messiness and ensures evenly sized muffins. For even easier scooping, spray the ice cream scoop with a little oil.

Using dark metal tins will produce muffins that have darker, firmer sides and that require shorter baking times. Light metal pans won't color the muffins as much; the muffins will take a bit longer to bake.

Muffin recipes always tell you to insert a toothpick or knife into the center of a muffin to see if it comes out clean, and my recipes are no exception. But what does "clean" mean? Simply that there shouldn't be any wet batter on the tester; it should come out dotted with a few dry crumbs or streaked with steam. Although toothpicks and butter knives are what I usually use, you can use all sorts of testing implements from a piece of spaghetti to an ice pick.

What is overmixing? Well, with muffins you want to get nice big crumbs. Mixing the batter too much can develop the gluten and make the muffin rubbery or gummy. So I mix using a fork, not a whisk or an electric mixer, and mix just until the dry ingredients are moistened, no more.

If you like big-ass muffin tops that spill over the sides, just fill the muffin tin almost to the rim and increase the baking time by 3 to 5 minutes. You'll only get ten muffins out of the batter instead of twelve, but you'll get those mountainous muffins that you so desire.

You might want to change the size of your muffins even further and branch out into jumbos or minis. No problem! For jumbos, increase the baking time between 7 and 10 minutes. And I've never met a mini that didn't bake in 12 to 15 minutes.

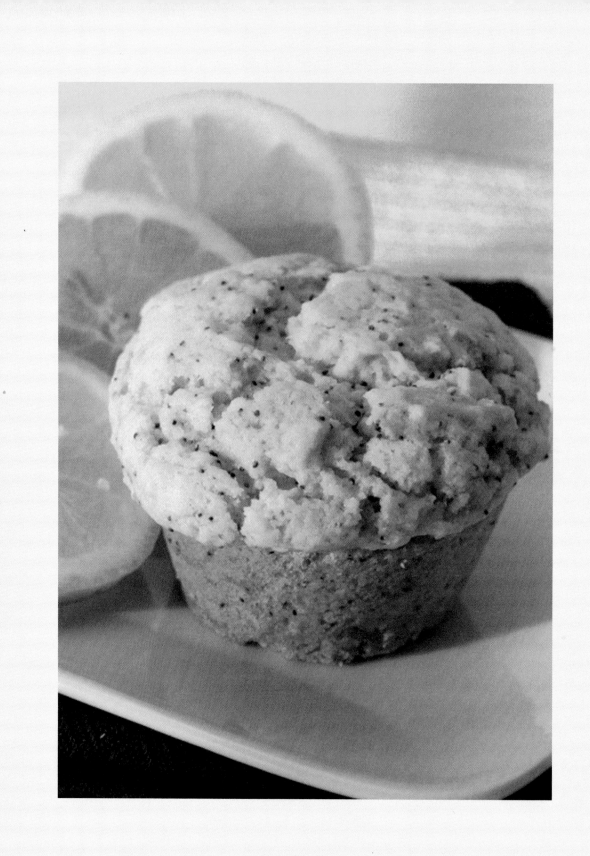

Lemon Poppy Seed Muffins

Makes 12 muffins

As ubiquitous as your pink-haired, lip-pierced, cat-tattoo barista, these muffins are a coffee shop staple. Who doesn't want to wake up to bright, fresh-tasting lemon?

2 cups all-purpose flour

²⁄₃ cup sugar

1 tablespoon baking powder

5 teaspoons poppy seeds

½ teaspoon salt

¾ cup soy milk (or almond milk, or rice milk)

¼ cup fresh lemon juice

½ cup canola oil

2 tablespoons lemon zest

2 teaspoons pure vanilla extract

Preheat the oven to 375°F. Lightly grease a muffin tin.

In a large mixing bowl, mix together flour, sugar, baking powder, poppy seeds, and salt. Make a well in the center and add milk, lemon juice, oil, zest, and vanilla. Mix just until all wet ingredients are moistened.

Fill the muffin tin three-quarters full and bake for 23 to 27 minutes, until muffins are lightly browned on top and a toothpick or knife inserted through the center comes out clean. When cool enough to handle, transfer to cooling racks to cool completely.

Bakery-Style Berry Muffins

Makes 12 muffins

I call these "bakery style" because they are those big, sweet, fluffy muffins that we find in bakery cafes these days. They're really more like dessert masquerading as breakfast, but who cares? I love to use frozen, mixed berries (raspberries, blueberries, and blackberries, usually) for maximum flavor, but you can use whatever kind of berries you like.

Preheat the oven to 375°F. Lightly grease a muffin tin.

In a large mixing bowl, stir together flour, sugar, baking powder, and salt. Make a well in the center and add the yogurt, milk, canola oil, and vanilla. Stir to combine. Fold in the berries.

Scoop the batter into the muffin tin; it should almost fill the entire tin. Bake for 26 to 30 minutes, or until a toothpick or butter knife inserted through the center of the muffin comes out clean. Let cool for a few minutes in the tin, then transfer muffins to a cooling rack to cool completely.

2 cups all-purpose flour

¾ cup sugar

1 tablespoon baking powder

½ teaspoon salt

½ cup soy yogurt

½ cup almond milk (or your favorite nondairy milk)

½ cup canola oil

2 teaspoons pure vanilla extract

1½ cups frozen mixed berries

Cocoa Raspberry Muffins

Makes 12 muffins

If you have my other books you will know that I think chocolate loves raspberry and vice versa. This muffin is my '80s power ballad to that love, may we all raise our wine coolers in reverence. Actually, enjoy these muffins with a strong cup of coffee spiked with raspberry syrup. These muffins are just a touch sweet, so if you're looking for something a bit more dessertlike, add ⅓ cup chocolate chips.

Preheat the oven to 375°F. Lightly grease a muffin tin. Measure out the milk in a large measuring cup and add the vinegar. Set aside to curdle.

In a large mixing bowl, stir together flour, cocoa powder, sugar, baking powder, and salt. Make a well in the center and add the milk, oil, applesauce and extracts. Stir to combine. Fold in the berries.

Scoop the batter into the muffin tin until the batter is almost filled to the rim. Bake for 24 to 28 minutes, or until a toothpick or butter knife inserted through the center of a muffin comes out clean. Let cool for a few minutes in the tin before transferring muffins to a cooling rack to cool completely.

1 cup almond milk (or your favorite nondairy milk)
1 teaspoon apple cider vinegar

1½ cups all-purpose flour
⅓ cup unsweetened cocoa powder
½ cup sugar
2 teaspoons baking powder
¼ teaspoon salt
⅓ cup canola oil
2 tablespoons unsweetened applesauce
1 teaspoon pure vanilla extract
¼ teaspoon almond extract

1½ cups raspberries

TIP Cocoa powder makes muffins more tender, so handle these with care. Don't rip them out of the muffin tins like there's no tomorrow; let them cool a bit and then gently coax them out.

Cranberry Orange Nut Muffins

Makes 12 muffins

Glorious orange muffins, studded with bright red cranberries and nummy pecans. A little almond extract really elevates the orange flavor, and the sweetness of the orange juice gives these a shiny, caramelized top.

Preheat the oven to 375°F. Lightly grease a muffin tin.

In a large mixing bowl, mix together flour, sugar, baking powder, baking soda, and salt. Make a well in the center and add orange juice, oil, zest, and extracts. Mix just until all wet ingredients are moistened. About halfway through mixing add the cranberries and nuts.

Fill the muffin tin three-quarters full and bake for 23 to 27 minutes, until muffins are lightly browned on top and a toothpick or knife inserted through the center comes out clean. When cool enough to handle, transfer the muffins to cooling racks to cool completely.

2 cups all-purpose flour
⅔ cup sugar
2 teaspoons baking powder
½ teaspoon baking soda
½ teaspoon salt

1 cup fresh orange juice
½ cup canola oil
2 tablespoons orange zest
2 teaspoons pure vanilla extract
¼ teaspoon almond extract

1½ cups fresh cranberries, roughly chopped
1 cup pecans, roughly chopped (walnut would be good, too)

TIP Cranberries are a bit of a pain to chop, what with their round shape and smooth exterior. They just love to jump around when you try to slice them. You can either pulse them just a few times in a food processor, or if using a chef's knife, place a handful at a time on the cutting board and, keeping the tip of the knife on the board, rock your knife back and forth very gently over the berries.

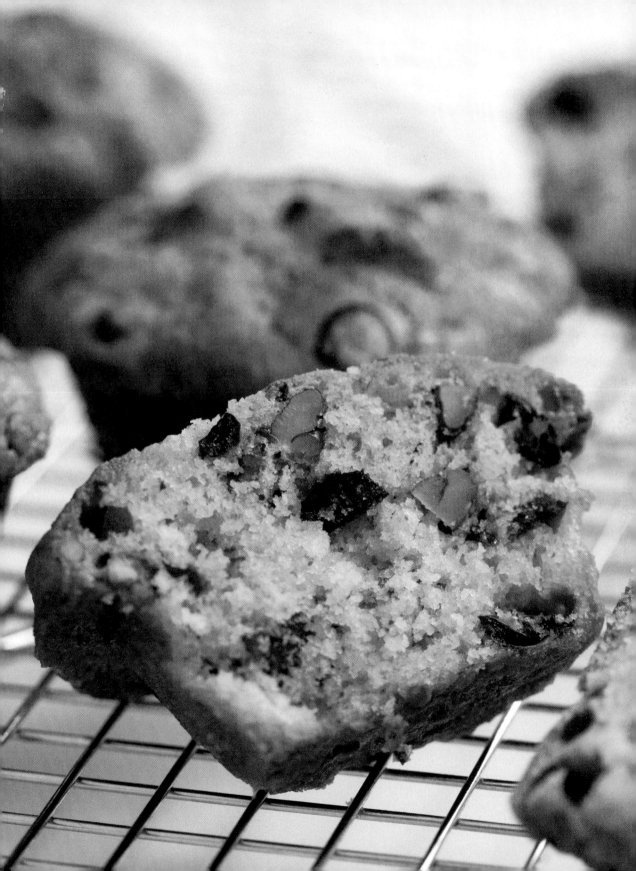

Toasted Coconut and Mango Muffins

Makes 12 muffins

Go on a tropical adventure with these muffins, unless you already live in the tropics, in which case stay put. Toasting the coconut really brings out its flavor, while dried mango adds little surprises of tangy sweetness. This recipe is a great introduction to white whole wheat flour, but if you don't have any or can't find it, you can use a mix of white flour and whole wheat flour.

Preheat the oven to 375°F. Lightly grease a muffin tin.

First, toast the coconut. Preheat a large pan over medium-low heat. Pour in the coconut and, using a spatula, move it around slowly and consistently for about 4 minutes. The coconut should start browning almost immediately; if it doesn't then turn the heat up just a bit. Remove from heat when toasted (it should appear honey brown to dark chestnut in color).

Measure milk into a measuring cup and add vinegar. Set aside to curdle.

In a large bowl, mix together flour, sugar, salt, baking powder, nutmeg, and allspice. Create a well in the center and add the milk mixture, oil, and extracts. Mix together until just combined, then fold in toasted coconut and mango. Fill the muffin tin three-quarters of the way with batter and bake for 23 to 27 minutes, until a knife or toothpick inserted through the center

1¼ cups unsweetened shredded coconut

1¼ cups almond milk (or your favorite nondairy milk)

1 teaspoon apple cider vinegar

1¾ cups white whole wheat flour
or 1 cup whole wheat flour and ¾ cup white flour

¼ cup sugar

¼ cup light brown sugar

½ teaspoon salt

1 tablespoon baking powder

½ teaspoon ground nutmeg

¼ teaspoon ground allspice

⅓ cup canola oil

1 teaspoon pure vanilla extract

1 teaspoon coconut extract (optional; you can also use another teaspoon vanilla)

¾ cup chopped dried mango (pieces should be pea-size or thereabouts)

comes out clean. Let cool a bit until you can loosen the muffins and transfer them to cooling racks to cool the rest of the way.

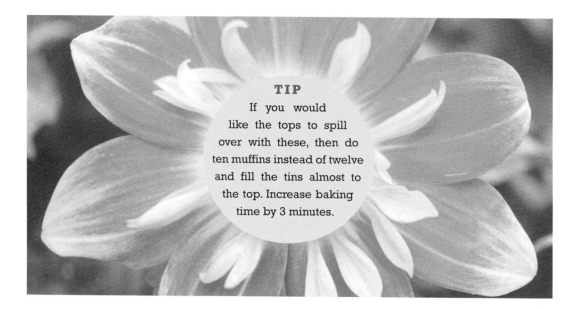

TIP
If you would like the tops to spill over with these, then do ten muffins instead of twelve and fill the tins almost to the top. Increase baking time by 3 minutes.

❊ VARIATIONS ❊

TOASTED COCONUT CHOCOLATE CHIP MUFFINS
Replace the dried mango with **1 cup chocolate chips**.

FRESH MANGO MUFFINS
Replace the dried mango with **2 cups diced fresh mango**.

Pumpkin Bran Muffins

Makes 12 muffins

Gone is that boring old bran muffin that your grandma took to synagogue every Saturday. Okay, so that muffin was pretty good. But these pumpkin ones are even better. Although this batter is really thick, the muffin comes out surprisingly light, with warm hints of cinnamon, ginger, and friends. If you like, fold in a cup of chopped walnuts.

Preheat the oven to 400°F. Lightly grease a muffin tin.

In a medium mixing bowl, mix together the pumpkin puree, milk, vinegar, oil, wheat bran, molasses, and vanilla for about a minute. You want to get the bran flakes well incorporated.

Separately, in a large mixing bowl, combine the flour, sugar, baking powder, salt, and spices. Make a well in the center and add the wet ingredients. Using a fork, gently stir together just until the dry ingredients are moistened, but be careful not to overmix since pumpkin likes to make batters gummy.

Fill the muffin tin three-quarters full. Bake for 25 to 27 minutes, or until a toothpick or butter knife inserted through the center of a muffin comes out clean. Let cool a bit until you can transfer the muffins to cooling racks to cool the rest of the way.

1 cup canned pumpkin or pumpkin puree

½ cup almond milk (or nondairy milk of your choice)

1 teaspoon apple cider vinegar

½ cup canola oil

1 cup wheat bran flakes (not bran cereal)

2 tablespoons molasses

2 teaspoons pure vanilla extract

1½ cups all-purpose flour or whole wheat pastry flour

¾ cup sugar

1 tablespoon baking powder

½ teaspoon salt

1 teaspoon ground cinnamon

1 teaspoon ground ginger

¼ teaspoon ground nutmeg

¼ teaspoon ground allspice

⅛ teaspoon ground cloves

Coffee Chip Muffins

Makes 12 muffins

I don't think I need to make the tough sell here: who doesn't love chocolate and coffee in the morning? These are the perfect brunch muffin, making good use of instant coffee instead of sometimes hard-to-find coffee extract.

Preheat the oven to 375°F. Lightly grease a muffin tin.

In a large measuring cup, measure out ½ cup of the milk. Stir in the coffee crystals and mix to dissolve. (A few undissolved crystals are okay.) Stir in the rest of the milk and the vinegar and set aside.

In a large mixing bowl, stir together the flour, sugar, baking powder, and salt. Make a well in the center and add the milk mixture, oil, and vanilla. Mix together until the batter is just moistened, being careful not to overmix. Fold in the chocolate chips.

Use an ice cream scoop to drop the batter into the muffin tin, filling it about three-quarters full. Bake for 22 to 26 minutes, until a knife or toothpick inserted through the center of a muffin comes out clean. Let cool a bit until you can remove the muffins and transfer them to cooling racks to cool the rest of the way.

1 cup almond milk (or your favorite nondairy milk)

1 heaping tablespoon instant coffee crystals

1 teaspoon apple cider vinegar

2 cups all-purpose flour

½ cup sugar

1 tablespoon baking powder

½ teaspoon salt

½ cup canola oil

1 teaspoon pure vanilla extract

½ cup chocolate chips

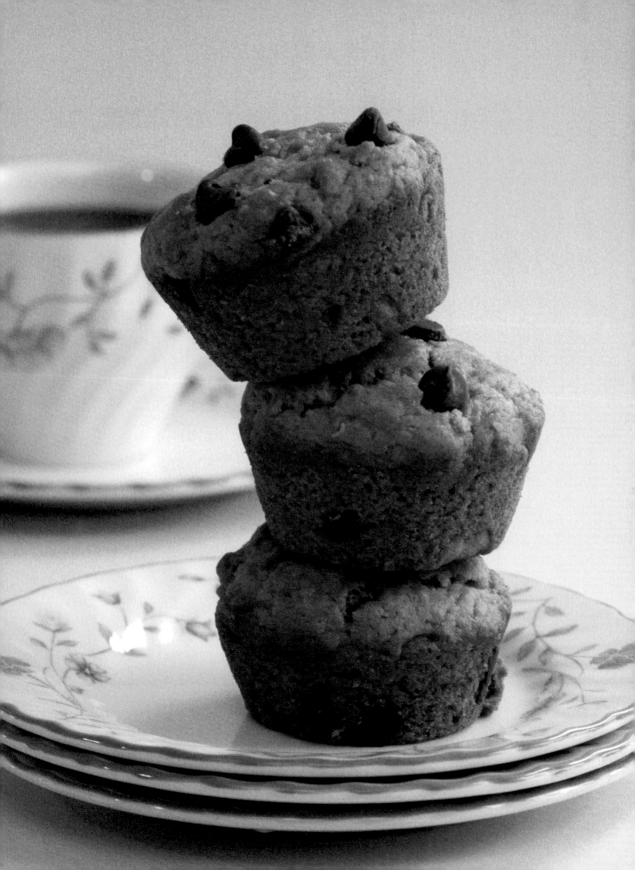

Zucchini Spelt Muffins

Makes 12 muffins

I like my zucchini muffins unobstructed—no nuts, no raisins, thank you very much. Just pure zucchini goodness with a few sweet spices gets me excited. And since you're already baking a muffin with a vegetable in it, why not go the extra healthy step and include some ground flax seeds for Omega-3s and spelt flour instead of white? P.S.—Just 'cause I don't like raisins doesn't mean you have to neglect them. If you like, add a cup for some extra sweetness.

Preheat the oven to 350°F. Lightly grease a muffin tin.

Combine the milk and ground flax seeds in a measuring cup and mix vigorously with a fork. Mix in the vinegar and set aside to curdle.

In a large mixing bowl, stir together the flour, baking powder, baking soda, salt, and spices. Make a well in the center and add the milk mixture, canola oil, brown sugar, and vanilla. Stir to combine. Fold in the zucchini.

Use an ice cream scoop to pour the batter into the muffin tin; it should almost fill the entire tin. Bake for 25 to 28 minutes, until the muffin tops are firm. A knife or toothpick inserted through a muffin may still come out steamy, because of the zucchinis, but it's still worth testing to make sure no batter is sticking. Zucchini makes these muffins so moist, be sure to let them cool in the tins for at least 20 minutes before removing them so that the tops don't break off. Transfer the muffins to a wire rack to cool completely.

1 cup almond milk (or your favorite nondairy milk)

3 tablespoons ground flax seeds

1 teaspoon apple cider vinegar

2½ cups spelt flour (see spelt tip page 171)

1 teaspoon baking powder

1 teaspoon baking soda

½ teaspoon salt

2 teaspoons ground cinnamon

½ teaspoon ground allspice

¼ teaspoon ground nutmeg

⅓ cup canola oil

½ cup packed light brown sugar

1 teaspoon pure vanilla extract

2 cups grated zucchini (about 1 pound or 2 small zucchinis)

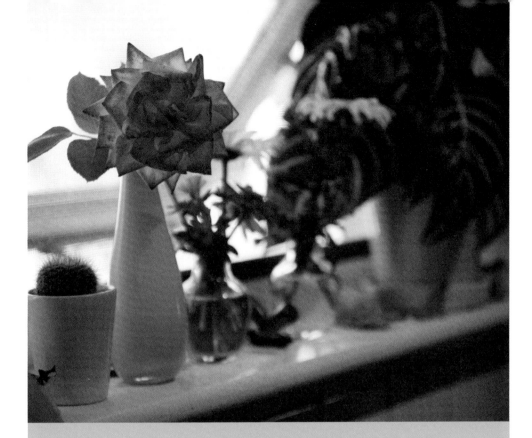

Spelt Flour: Spelting It Out for You

Not only is spelt great for making puns, it's also wonderful for baking. It gives baked goods a delightfully rustic and crumbly crumb that is especially well suited for muffins. The taste is a bit more wholesome than what you get with white flour—nuttier and more wheaty. Spelt is an ancestor of wheat (you could call it an "heirloom" wheat if you wanted to sound refined), but its lower gluten content makes it easier to work with since you don't have to worry as much about overmixing spelt batter. As with most whole-grain flours, I think it's best to let spelt muffins cool completely before taking a bite; this lets the flavors mellow out and lose some of their "healthfoodiness." Some of my testers disagreed, though, and just ate them right out of the muffin tins. Savages.

East Coast Coffee Cake

Serves 8

In NYC, coffee cake has no coffee in it, which can be confusing. But here's what we're talking about: a rich, moist, yellow cake topped with a thick and messy crumb topping, perfect for serving with coffee. I'm going to give you the basic recipe, but I recommend trying one of the variations. Maybe something sophisticated like cinnamon fig, or something sweet and snacky like chocolate chip. You can even get crazy and combine the chocolate chip with a fruit variation, like raspberry. I really like to bake this in a round springform pan, but an 8-inch brownie pan will work, too.

Preheat the oven to 375°F. Lightly grease an 8-inch round springform pan or 8-inch square pan. Measure out the milk for the cake and mix in the teaspoon of vinegar; set aside to curdle. Then begin preparing the topping.

MAKE THE TOPPING

In a small mixing bowl, mix together the flour, sugar, cinnamon, and nutmeg. Drizzle in the canola oil by the tablespoonful (you can eyeball it, no reason to whip out a tablespoon). Use your fingers to swish around the mixture until crumbs form. Alternate swishing and adding canola oil until all the oil is used and large crumbs have formed. Some of the topping is still going to be sandy and that's fine, just so long as you have mostly nice big crumbs. You can add another table-

For the topping:

1 cup all-purpose flour

⅓ cup brown sugar

1 teaspoon ground cinnamon

¼ teaspoon ground nutmeg

¼ cup canola oil, plus up to 2 tablespoons more if needed

For the cake:

¾ cup soy milk (or any nondairy milk)

1 teaspoon apple cider vinegar

⅓ cup sugar

½ cup canola oil

1 teaspoon pure vanilla extract

1¼ cups all-purpose flour

2 teaspoons baking powder

½ teaspoon salt

For serving:

2 tablespoons powdered sugar (optional)

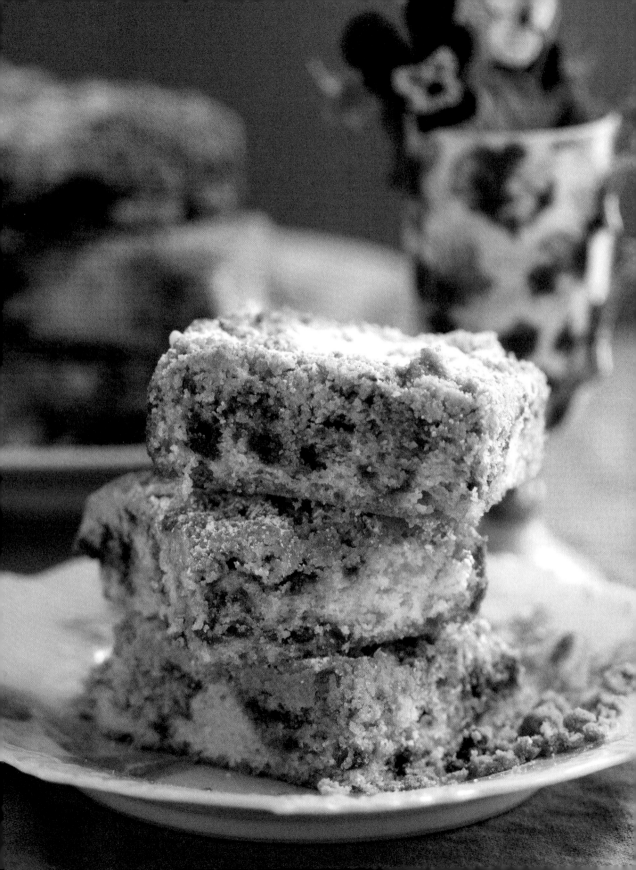

spoon or two of oil if needed; it seems to vary for me how much I use and if there's a reason I can't tell you why.

MAKE THE CAKE

In a large mixing bowl, mix together the milk mixture, sugar, canola oil, and vanilla. Sift in the flour, baking powder, and salt and mix until smooth.

Pour the cake batter into the prepared pan. Evenly sprinkle on the topping and pat it down just a bit. Bake for 35 to 40 minutes, or until a knife inserted through the center comes out clean.

Let cool for at least an hour before slicing and serving. Sift optional powdered sugar over the top once cooled.

※ VARIATIONS ※

CINNAMON FIG

This is a yummy option for a layer of sticky figginess between the cake and the crumb topping. Finely chop **1½ cups dried mission figs** into pea-size pieces. Mix with **1 teaspoon ground cinnamon** and **2 tablespoons brown sugar**. After pouring the cake batter into the pan, layer on the figs. Add the crumb topping and pat down lightly.

CHOCOLATE CHIP

You can do this two ways—each has its charms. One is to fold **1 cup chocolate chips** into the cake batter. The other is to sprinkle **1 cup chocolate chips** on top of the batter before adding the crumb topping. This way you have a layer of chocolate between the cake and the crumbs. The second option is great for using in conjunction with other cake variations.

BERRY

You can use whatever berry is in season to brighten up any brunch spread. Fold **1 cup fresh berries** into the batter. If using frozen, then make sure they are frozen, not thawed, when you stir them in and increase baking time by 5 minutes. **A teaspoon citrus zest** is wonderful with the berry option, but not entirely necessary.

RASPBERRY CHOCOLATE

If you haven't noticed yet, I kill for raspberry and chocolate. But it's the good kind of killing, the kind that gets me raspberries and chocolate. Add **1 cup raspberries** into the cake batter (see above) and layer **1¼ cups chocolate chips** on top of the cake batter before adding the crumb topping.

BANANA

You can use this option in conjunction with any of the other variations if you want to up the ante with a little banana goodness. Just mash up **1 banana** and add it to the wet ingredients of the batter. Also, add an additional **2 tablespoons flour**.

APRICOT CARDAMOM

Feeling a little Turkish? Finely chop **1½ cups dried apricots** into pea-size pieces. Mix with **½ teaspoon ground cardamom** and **2 tablespoons brown sugar**. Also, add **½ teaspoon cardamom** to the crumb topping. After pouring the cake batter into the pan, layer on the apricots. Add the crumb topping and pat down lightly.

JAM SWIRL

A fun and swirly variation that doesn't take hardly any extra work. Well, besides fishing around in your fridge for that jar of jam that's just gotta be in there. Get **¾ cup of your favorite jam**. Splotch all over the batter with spoonfuls of jam and use a knife to swirl into the batter. Add the crumb topping and pat down lightly.

Pain au Chocolat

Makes 8 pastries

Pain au Chocolat is a flaky bread (that's *pain* to you, Monsieur) filled with, you guessed it, chocolate! But we lazy Americans have figured out a way to skip those years of patisserie apprenticeship to learn how to make a nice, flaky pastry. Instead, we're just using layers of phyllo stuffed with chocolate chips and fresh fruit of our choice. Don't be mad at us, France! Be mad at the Greeks! This comes together super-duper fast and bakes in only 15 minutes.

Preheat the oven to 350°F.

Brush a sheet of phyllo with oil. Layer on 3 more sheets, brushing each with oil. Put 2 tablespoons of chocolate chips about 3 inches from the left-hand side and 1 inch from the bottom. Place the fruit over the chocolate chips. Fold the bottom up, then fold the top down to cover the chocolate chips and fruit. Brush with oil, then fold the left flap over and roll like a burrito. Brush with oil on the bottom and place on baking sheet. Continue with the remaining Pain au Chocolats. Brush tops with oil; bake for 15 minutes or until golden brown.

Remove from the oven and transfer to cooling racks. They taste so good when they're still a bit warm and all melty, but don't try when they are still hot or you'll burn your tongue. There are worse ways to die than burned chocolate tongue, but still, wait like half an hour.

1 pound phyllo dough, thawed

1 cup chocolate chips

½ cup canola oil

Fruit choices (mix and match or choose one of the following; do not overstuff these!):

Strawberries, sliced in half (two halves per serving)

Banana, sliced on the bias (one slice per serving)

Raspberries (use three berries per serving)

Pear, thinly sliced (one slice per serving)

Pineapple (half a ring per serving)

TIP If you've never worked with phyllo before here are some things you should know:

You'll find it in the frozen section of your supermarket.

It needs to thaw completely before using. Place it in the fridge to thaw at least overnight; if you leave it out on the counter it gets soggy and sticks.

Once thawed, let it rest on the counter for around 20 minutes for best results. When it's at room temperature, it's less moist and thus has less chance of ripping.

If you do tear a sheet, don't sweat it too bad. Either use the torn sheet as one of the inside ones or scrap it. This recipe calls for a little more phyllo than needed, just in case disaster strikes.

Have everything for your recipe prepared and ready to go before beginning to work with the phyllo. I don't say that to scare you, just to minimize the chances that your phyllo will dry out. If it's taking you a while to make these or if you need to step away, cover the unwrapped phyllo.

This recipe calls for 9 x 14-inch sheets of phyllo, which is a standard size. However, if your sheets are larger, you may need to slice them in half with a knife to get the right size. Just take a sharp knife and slice a few at a time down the middle with the tip of the knife.

Cinnamon Rolls

Makes 12 rolls

Is there anything better than coming out of the cold into a warm kitchen and inhaling a blast of cinnamon air? Don't answer that, because there simply isn't. If you want to be loved, bake cinnamon rolls. It takes a little time and patience but guess what? The payoff is … cinnamon rolls!

In a large mixing bowl, dissolve the yeast and 1 teaspoon sugar in the water. Let sit for a few minutes. Add the rest of the sugar, milk, oil, salt, cinnamon, and 2 cups of flour. Stir for about a minute. Add flour by the ½ cupfuls until you have added about 3½ cups. Knead to form a soft dough; if it's sticky then add flour until it is no longer sticky.

Lightly flour a clean, flat surface and knead dough for 5 minutes, or until nice and smooth. Place in a greased bowl (about 2 teaspoons canola oil should do it), turn to coat, cover with a towel or plastic wrap and let rise in a warmish place until doubled in size, about an hour.

Once dough has risen, punch it down and let it rest for about 10 minutes. In the meantime, prepare the filling by mixing all the ingredients together.

Lightly flour a work surface again and stretch and roll the dough out into a rectangle that's about 12 by 18 inches. Sprinkle the filling evenly over the surface of the dough and dot with the margarine. Just break the margarine into small pieces with your fingers; it doesn't have to be too precise.

For the dough:

1 packet active dry yeast (2¼ teaspoons)

⅓ cup sugar, plus 1 teaspoon

½ cup lukewarm water

¾ cup milk, at room temperature

⅓ cup canola oil

¾ teaspoon salt

1 teaspoon ground cinnamon

3½ to 4 cups flour

For the filling:

¼ cup brown sugar

¼ cup regular sugar

1 tablespoon ground cinnamon

2 tablespoons flour

To roll:

¼ cup nonhydrogenated margarine

For the icing:

1 cup powdered sugar

1½ to 2 tablespoons almond milk (or your favorite nondairy milk)

1 teaspoon pure vanilla extract

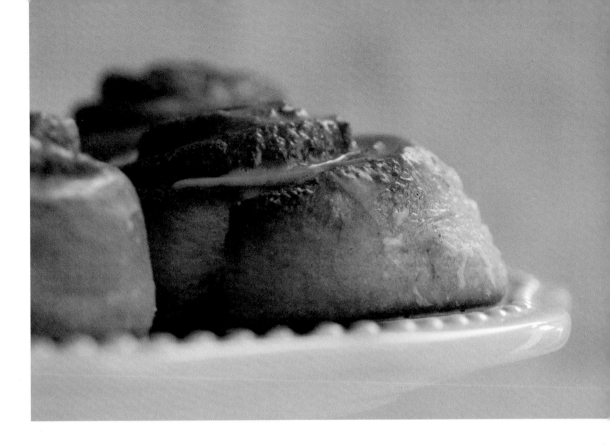

Firmly roll up from the long side. Go as slow as you need to get it as tight as you can. Use a little water to pinch the seam together to seal.

Lightly spray an 11 x 13-inch rimmed baking pan. Slice dough into twelve even pieces. Sometimes if my ends are too sloppy to deal with, I slice off about an inch and scrap it so that I have more even pieces. An easy way to make twelve slices is to first cut into quarters and then cut each quarter into thirds.

Place in a baking pan cut side down; they'll be pretty snug. You might lose some of the sugar mixture, but don't sweat it. Cover with a towel and let rise for 30 to 45 minutes; the rolls should look not quite doubled in size.

Preheat the oven to 375°F. Bake for 18 to 22 minutes; when ready they should look lightly browned and puffy. Remove from the oven. Prepare the icing by mixing all the ingredients together with a fork in a small mixing bowl. Use 1½ tablespoons of liquid at first, adding another ½ tablespoon if needed.

Drizzle the icing over the warm cinnamon buns and serve as soon as you can!

Scones

Makes 12 scones

This is the quintessential scone: a little bit of crunch on the outside, a moist, almost flaky interior, not too sweet flavor, and perfect for a spot of jam or a pat of vegan butter. You don't have to craft these into triangles, just drop them onto the baking sheet with a measuring spoon instead. Easy! Check out the variations and come up with some scone creations of your own.

Preheat the oven to 375°F. Lightly grease a baking sheet or line it with parchment paper. Measure out the milk in a large measuring cup and add the vinegar to it. Set aside to curdle.

Combine the flour, baking powder, salt, and sugar in a large mixing bowl. Add the shortening in small clumps, then use your fingers or a pastry cutter to cut it into the flour until the dough texture becomes pebblelike. (You can also use a food processor for this step, but I prefer to use my hands because it's faster and means less to clean up afterwards.)

Create a well in the center and add the milk mixture, oil, and vanilla. Mix with a wooden spoon until about half of the flour is incorporated. Mix again until all the ingredients are just moistened, taking care not to overmix. A couple of dry-looking spots are just fine.

Spray a ¼-cup measuring cup with cooking spray and use the cup to scoop the scones onto the baking sheet.

1¼ cups almond milk (or your favorite nondairy milk)

2 teaspoons apple cider vinegar

3 cups flour

2 tablespoons baking powder

½ teaspoon salt

½ cup sugar, plus extra for sprinkling

½ cup nonhydrogenated vegetable shortening

2 tablespoons canola oil

1 teaspoon pure vanilla extract

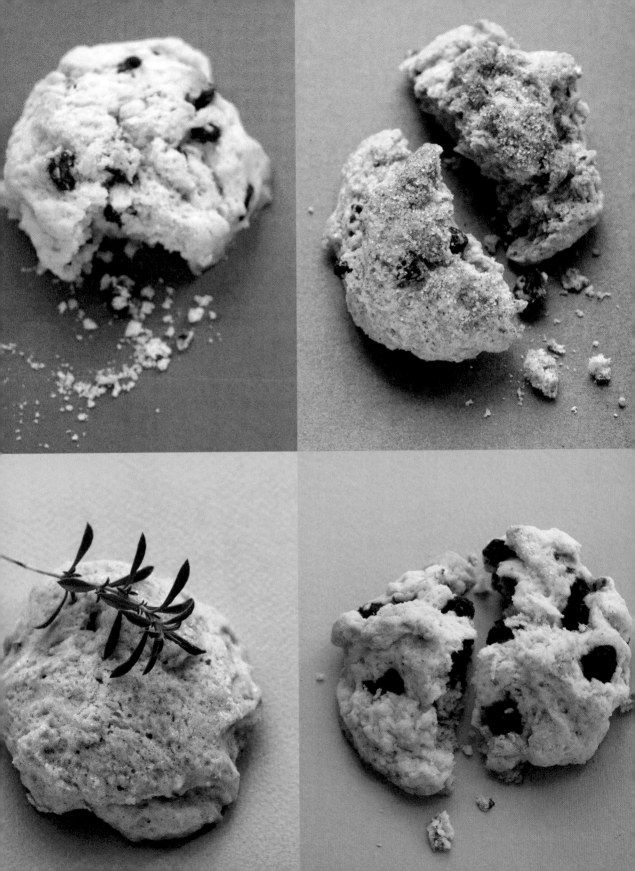

Dust the tops of the scones with more sugar, then bake for 18 to 22 minutes, until tops are lightly browned and firm to the touch. Transfer the scones to a cooling rack to cool (but I think they taste best still slightly warm).

☼ VARIATIONS ☼

Scones Are a Window to the Soul

The scone is really the perfect canvas for your culinary creativity. This is one of my favorite recipes to play around with and use fresh and seasonal ingredients (or whatever is around the house). Here are some of my favorite variations, but I also hope you'll come up with some great new variations, too.

BERRY SCONES

For berry scones, blueberry is a popular choice. Fold **2 cups fresh or frozen blueberries** into the dough about halfway through mixing. You can take a cue from the Blueberry Ginger Spelt Muffins (page 155) and add **1½ tablespoons ground ginger**, too. One of my favorite berry combinations is marionberry and lavender. Marionberries are big, juicy, floral-tasting berries that are just begging for a delicate pairing. Here in Portland the berry-picking farms are side by side with the lavender farms. The fragrance will send you running through the fields like a romance novel. For this effect, in addition to the berries, add **¼ cup chopped culinary lavender** to the dry ingredients.

CHOCOLATE CHIP SCONES

Chocolate chips are always a game changer. After lightly mixing the batter, fold in **1 cup chocolate chips**. You can mix chocolate and berries, too (just reduce the amount of berries to 1½ cups). Another favorite combo of mine is ginger and chocolate: add **½ cup chopped crystallized ginger**.

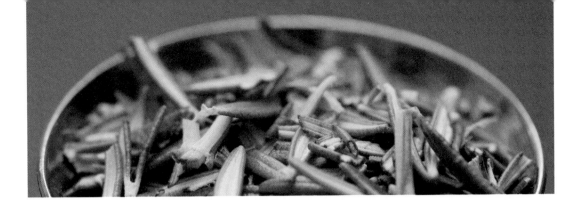

APPLE ROSEMARY SCONES

There's a scone sold in Portland made with apples and rosemary that I've become a bit addicted to. Fold in **1½ cups diced apple**. Add **¼ cup finely chopped fresh rosemary (or 2 tablespoons dried)** to the dry ingredients, as well as **¼ teaspoon ground nutmeg** and **1 teaspoon ground cinnamon**. If not using the rosemary, up the cinnamon to 2 teaspoons and add **a pinch of cloves**.

RAISINS AND SPICE SCONES

I love this combo during the winter holidays when I'm (oh, the horror!) sick of pumpkin baked goods. Add **1 cup raisins, 2 teaspoons cinnamon, 1 teaspoon allspice, ½ teaspoon ground nutmeg, and ¼ teaspoon cloves**. Also, mix together **2 tablespoons sugar** and **1 teaspoon cinnamon** and sprinkle that over the scones before baking.

Tomato Rosemary Scones

Makes 12 scones

A fragrant savory scone that's a pretty orange color and flecked with fresh rosemary. They are sure to class up the joint. I love the olive-y notes from the olive oil, but if you're a cheapskate, use canola oil.

3 cups all-purpose flour

2 tablespoons baking powder

¼ cup sugar

½ teaspoon salt

½ teaspoon ground black pepper

⅓ cup olive oil

1 fourteen-ounce can tomato sauce (about 1½ cups)

1 teaspoon apple cider vinegar

2 tablespoons fresh chopped rosemary (about 4 sprigs worth)

Preheat the oven to 400°F. Lightly grease a baking sheet.

In a large mixing bowl, combine the flour, baking powder, sugar, salt, and pepper.

Measure the olive oil into a large measuring cup (3 cups or larger) and whisk in the tomato sauce, vinegar, and rosemary. You can mix it all directly in the measuring cup, so you don't have to dirty up another dish.

Make a well in the center of the flour and add the wet ingredients. Gently mix, using a wooden spoon. Once the batter is loosely holding together, lightly flour a clean work surface and turn your dough onto it. Gently knead until a soft dough forms; it's important not to overmix it or it will become gummy. (To give you an idea of what it should look like, some patches of flour are great.) If the dough seems sticky, add a little flour as you knead, until it's easier to work with.

Divide dough in two and form each section into a 6-inch disk. Slice each disk into six pieces, like a pizza pie. (To do this, cut in half and then cut each half into thirds.) Place scones on a baking sheet and bake for 14 to 16 minutes; the tops should be firm. Remove the scones from the oven and let cool a bit on a plate or cooling rack. Serve either warm or at room temperature.

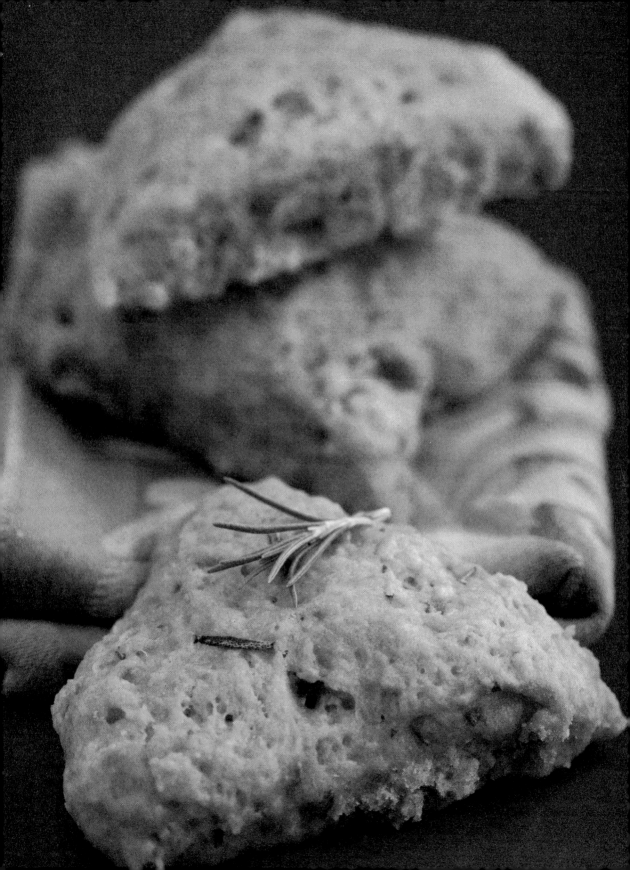

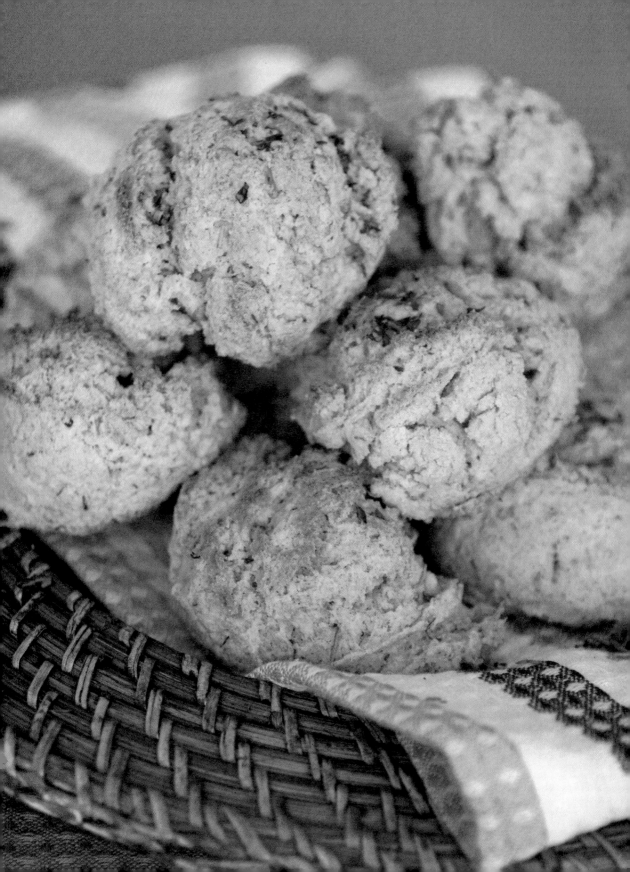

Herbed Whole Wheat Drop Biscuits

Makes 12 biscuits

I don't know, I can't be bothered to do "cut-out" biscuits anymore. It just seems silly when you can drop 'em on the pan with much less fuss. But enough of my biscuit pathos. These whole wheat biscuits are slightly more crumbly than traditional white flour biscuits. They have a pleasant, crunchy bite that I can get down with, plus they're just perfect for sopping up gravy. However, if you like, you can substitute all-purpose flour for whole wheat.

Preheat the oven to 450°F. Grease a baking sheet.

In a large bowl, mix together the flour, baking powder, herbs, and salt. Cut the shortening and margarine into the flour using your fingers or a pastry knife, or two knives held together, until pebble-to-marble-size pieces of dough form. Add the milk and use a wooden spoon to combine into a soft dough.

Use an ice cream scoop or ¼-cup measuring cup to scoop biscuits onto the baking sheet. Bake for 15 to 18 minutes, until the biscuits are lightly browned. Transfer the biscuits to a cooling rack but serve warm if you can.

2 cups whole wheat pastry flour

5 teaspoons baking powder

2 teaspoons dried thyme

2 teaspoons dried rosemary

1 teaspoon salt

3 tablespoons cold nonhydrogenated vegetable shortening

2 tablespoons cold nonhydrogenated margarine

1 cup almond milk (or your favorite nondairy milk)

Chive Spelt Mini-Biscuits

Makes 18 biscuits

Okay, seriously, I know many recipes say that their subject is addictive, but these mini-biscuits really, really are. They're flaky, loaded with chives, and have that nice, toasty taste. Serve them with scrambled tofu and gravy and try not to eat 20 million.

Note: These depend on vinegar and baking soda for their leavening; don't worry that there's no baking powder in the recipe! It's not a typo.

½ cup almond milk (or your favorite nondairy milk)

1 tablespoon apple cider vinegar

2 cups spelt flour (see spelt tip page 171)

2 teaspoons baking soda

½ teaspoon salt

½ cup nonhydrogenated vegetable shortening

¾ cup finely chopped chives

1 tablespoon agave nectar or pure maple syrup

2 tablespoons olive oil

Preheat the oven to 375°F. Lightly grease a baking sheet. Measure the milk in a large measuring cup and add the vinegar. Set aside to curdle.

In a large mixing bowl, mix together the spelt, baking soda, and salt. Now you're going to get your hands dirty. Drop half the shortening into the flour in pieces and mix using your fingers. Add the rest of the shortening and now really get it mixed in there, until the dough looks like pebbly crumbs. (This method really beats using a pastry cutter. And if you're using spelt flour, you're not really in danger of overmixing because of its low gluten content.)

Mix the chives into the dough. Meanwhile, add the agave and oil to the milk mixture, then pour it into the flour and use a fork to mix just until the dough is moistened.

Use a tablespoon to scoop the dough into rounded biscuits and place on a baking sheet about 2 inches apart. Bake for 13 to 15 minutes. When ready, the biscuits should look a bit darker and be firm to the touch. Let cool for a few minutes but serve warm if you can.

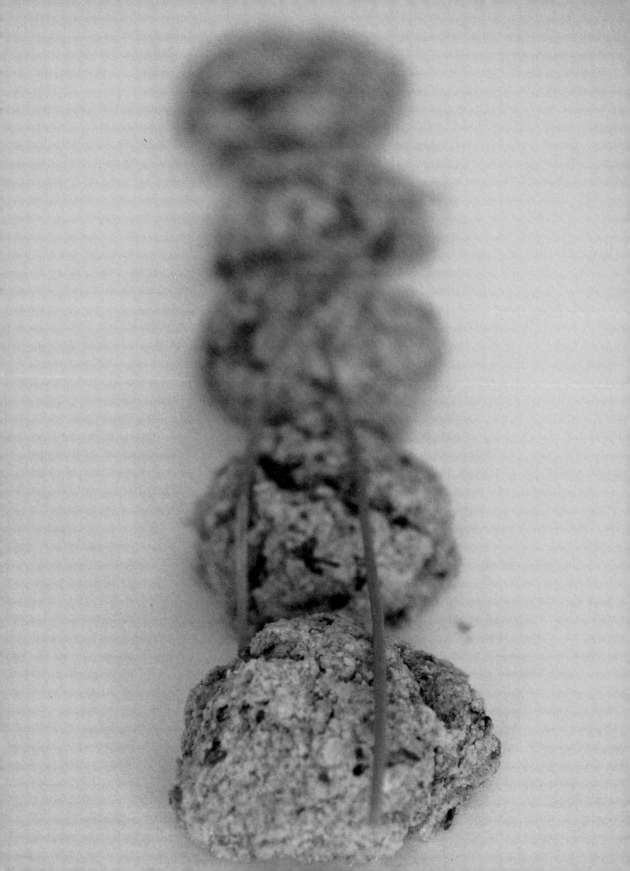

English Muffins

Makes 8 muffins

These are really fun to make. Bread dough is made the normal way, then cut out into circles, briefly panfried, then baked until nice and puffy. Make these as a special treat for your brunch guests the night before. It is such a deeply satisfying feeling to watch the vegan butter melt into nooks and crannies that you baked all by yourself.

1 teaspoon active dry yeast

1 tablespoon sugar

1 cup lukewarm water

2¼ cups all-purpose flour

1¼ teaspoons salt

3 tablespoons nonhydrogenated margarine, room temperature

A few tablespoons cornmeal

Nonhydrogenated margarine for skillet

In a small bowl, combine the yeast, sugar, and water; set aside until the yeast has dissolved, about 5 minutes. In a large mixing bowl, combine the flour and salt; make a well in the center and add the yeast mixture and margarine. Mix until a dough forms, then turn out onto a floured surface; knead until smooth and springy, 6 to 10 minutes. Return the dough to the bowl and cover with plastic wrap or a damp tea towel; set in a warm place and let rise until just about doubled, about an hour.

Preheat a cookie sheet in the oven to 350°F. Punch dough down and knead for a minute, then roll out on a floured surface until ½ inch thick. Cut into 3-inch rounds using a cookie cutter and pat both sides into cornmeal. Preheat a large skillet, preferably cast iron, over medium heat; melt about 1 tablespoon margarine in it (the pan should not be hot enough to burn the margarine). Cook the muffins in the pan in small batches so as not to crowd the pan, flipping once, about 1 minute a side or until it looks lightly browned like an English muffin. Put each batch straight from the skillet into the oven; bake for 6 to 10 minutes. Cool on a wire rack for half an hour before serving.

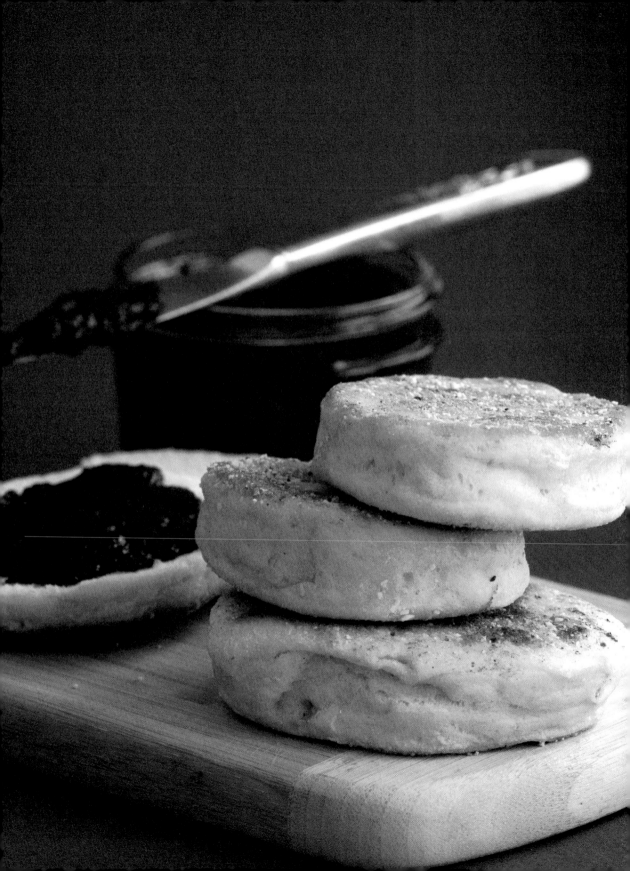

Cornbread Biscuits

Makes 20 to 22 biscuits

I t's cornbread ... but it's a biscuit. It's a cornbread biscuit. And it isn't messing around. Serve these alongside any of the Latin-themed brunches. Although these biscuits aren't overly sweet, you can reduce the sugar if you prefer your cornbread super savory. Just use 2 tablespoons of sugar and you are all set.

2 cups flour

1 cup stone-ground cornmeal

¼ cup sugar

2 tablespoons baking powder

½ teaspoon salt

⅓ cup canola oil

1 cup almond milk (or your favorite nondairy milk)

2 teaspoons apple cider vinegar

Preheat the oven to 400°F. Grease two baking sheets (or use one for two batches if your oven is too small and your baking sheet too large. But I don't advise placing the sheets on two oven racks as they need to heat evenly).

Combine the flour, cornmeal, sugar, baking powder, and salt in a large mixing bowl. Make a well in the center and pour in the oil, milk, and vinegar. Gently mix until all the ingredients are just moistened (some lumps of flour in the batter are just fine).

Use a tablespoon to dole out heaping spoonfuls of batter onto the baking sheets about 2 inches apart. Bake biscuits for 12 to 14 minutes, until the tops are firm. The bottoms should be lightly browned. They can cool on the baking sheet, no problem. Let them sit for about 10 minutes, then serve warm. They're good at room temp, too, though.

☼ VARIATION ☼

Add ¼ cup chopped seeded jalapeños for a spicy treat.

Bagels

Makes 12 bagels

Nothing beats a big, doughy, fresh-from-the-oven NYC bagel, but when you aren't in NYC these are a wonderful compromise. Bagels are boiled first and then baked, creating a beautiful glossy exterior and a soft, chewy interior. Serve with Garden Herb Spread (page 210) or doctor up some vegan cream cheese and serve with slices of salted tomatoes.

3 tablespoons sugar, divided
1½ cups lukewarm water
one ¼-ounce packet dry
   active yeast

4 cups all-purpose flour
2 tablespoons vital wheat gluten
2 teaspoons salt
Poppy seeds or sesame seeds
   (optional)

Vegetable oil for the rising bowl
Salt for the boiling water
   (2 teaspoons or so)

In a small mixing bowl, dissolve 1 tablespoon of the sugar in the water, then add the yeast. In a separate large mixing bowl mix together the other ingredients. Add the yeast mixture and knead for a good 10 minutes or so; the dough should be neither dry nor wet but nicely tacky. You can use a mixer with a dough hook for the kneading process, that works great. Place dough in an oiled bowl and cover with a damp cloth (or plastic wrap) and let sit for an hour or so. It won't rise a lot but it should be nicely springy.

Put a large pot of salted water on to boil and preheat the oven to 425°F. Turn dough out onto a dry surface and cut into 12 equal pieces. Roll each piece into a ball, then use your thumbs to tuck the dough under until you poke a hole through the center, then work the hole until it's roughly half-dollar size (about ¾ of an inch). If you would like to add poppy or sesame seeds, then place a thin layer of seeds on a plate and lightly pat each side of the bagel into the seeds. Place the bagels on a baking sheet covered with parchment, cover with a damp towel, and wait for the water to boil.

Once boiling, reduce to a gentle simmer and add three of the bagels—they should bob up to the surface in a few seconds; if they don't, nudge them with a spoon until they unstick. Simmer for one minute, then flip them over and simmer for another minute. Remove the bagels using a slotted spoon and place them back on the baking sheet. Repeat until all your bagels are boiled, then place in the oven. Bake for 18 to 20 minutes, until nice and amber brown, then remove and let sit for 30 minutes. The bagels are now ready.

Fun with Vegan Cream Cheese

I'm not crazy about vegan cream cheese recipes that invariably spell "cheese" in new and cute ways and usually tell you to blend up some tofu with vinegar. Yeah. No thanks. If I want a tofu spread I'll have a tofu spread (see Garden Herb Spread, page 210). If I want cream cheese, I'll just use that store-bought stuff that actually tastes good. But you don't have to just put the tub out and call your guests to the table. Instead, add some love to that bagel topper. Bagel shops all over NYC carry a variety of doctored-up vegan cream cheeses; hopefully the rest of the world will follow suit someday.

For all the following recipes, transfer the cream cheese to a mixing bowl, work the ingredients in with a fork, and then smooth cream cheese out with a spatula. For the best presentation, transfer to a nice small bowl to serve; don't just serve it out of the bowl it was mixed in. That's tacky.

SUNDRIED TOMATO

Rehydrate about ½ **cup chopped sundried tomatoes** in warm water for about ½ an hour. Mix into the cream cheese.

CHIPOTLE

Remove seeds from **2 or 3 canned chipotles in adobo sauce**. Mash chipotles up with a fork and mix into the cream cheese.

CARAMELIZED ONION

Prepare a ½ **recipe of the caramelized onions** in the Caramelized Vidalia Onion Quiche (page 43). Cool completely, then mix into the cream cheese.

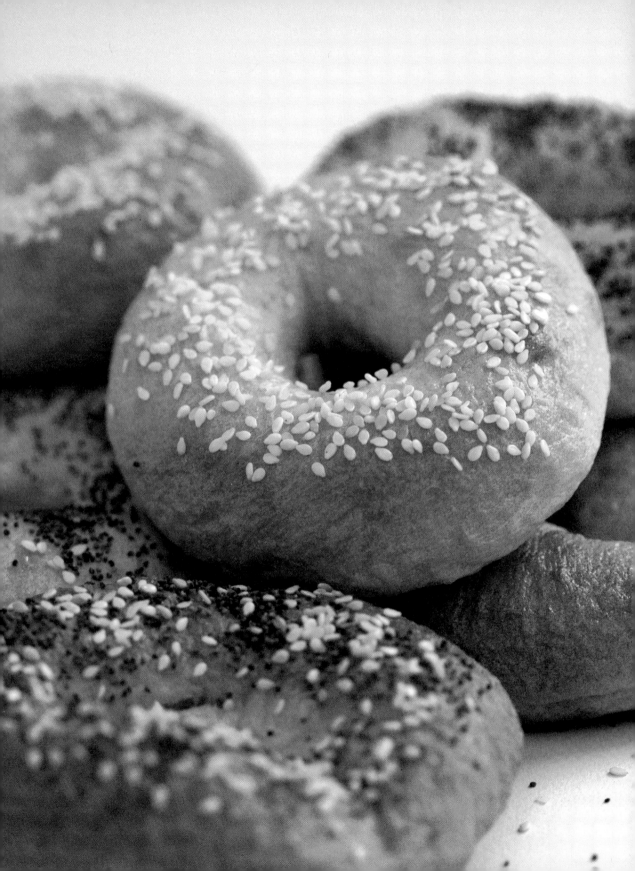

VEGETABLE

Mix in ¼ **cup each very finely chopped carrots, celery,** and **red bell pepper**.

SCALLION

Finely chop **a small bunch of scallions**. Mix into the cream cheese.

ONION CHIVE

Mix in ½ **cup finely chopped chive** plus **2 tablespoons onion powder**.

CINNAMON RAISIN

This sweet cream cheese topping is pretty popular in Brooklyn. Add **1 teaspoon ground cinnamon** and ½ **cup raisins**.

OLIVE

Mix in ½ **cup seeded, chopped olives**; try green olives, kalamata, oil cured, or a mix of all three.

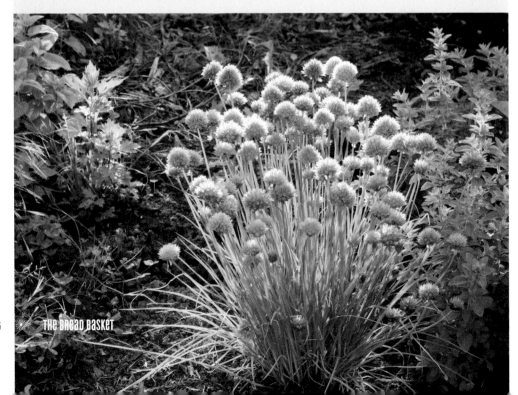

Poppy Seed Pull-Apart Rolls

Makes 16 rolls

Why make rolls that just sit around being rolls when you can make pull-apart rolls? I love these for the audience participation aspect, guests reaching in and claiming their little section in the breadbasket.

In a small bowl, combine the yeast, sugar, and water; set aside until the yeast dissolves, 5 minutes or so. In a large mixing bowl, combine the flours and salt; make a well in the center and add the yeast mixture. Mix until a dough forms, then turn out onto a floured surface; knead until smooth and springy, 6 to 10 minutes. Return the dough to the bowl and cover with plastic wrap or a damp tea towel; set in a warm place and let rise until roughly doubled, about an hour.

Grease a 9-inch cake pan. Punch down the risen dough; knead in the poppy seeds. Divide the dough into sixteen equal pieces and roll into balls; place them in the pan, first one right in the middle and then form rings of rolls around that one. Cover and let rise again, about and hour.

Preheat the oven to 375°F. Brush the tops of the rolls with oil, sprinkle on the remaining poppy seeds, and bake until golden brown on top, about 30 minutes. Let cool before serving.

1 teaspoon active dry yeast
1 tablespoon sugar
1¼ cups lukewarm water

1½ cups all-purpose flour
1½ cups whole wheat flour
2 teaspoons salt

¼ cup poppy seeds
Melted margarine or oil for glazing
2 tablespoons poppy seeds for sprinkling

The Toppings

Gravy, Sauces, and Spreads
to Mess Up Your Bib

Ginger Cranberry Sauce

Makes 3 cups

This is a perfect topping for the Pumpkin Pancakes (page 85) or any winter holiday brunch.

2 cups fresh cranberries

1¼ cups water

⅓ cup sugar

1 tablespoon grated fresh ginger

¼ cup pure maple syrup

Mix together cranberries, water, and sugar in a saucepan. Cover and bring to a boil. Lower the heat a bit and let simmer for about 10 minutes. Uncover and let simmer until the mixture is reduced by about half, 10 more minutes or so. Remove from heat and grate in the ginger. Let cool for at least half an hour and stir in the maple syrup. Serve warm.

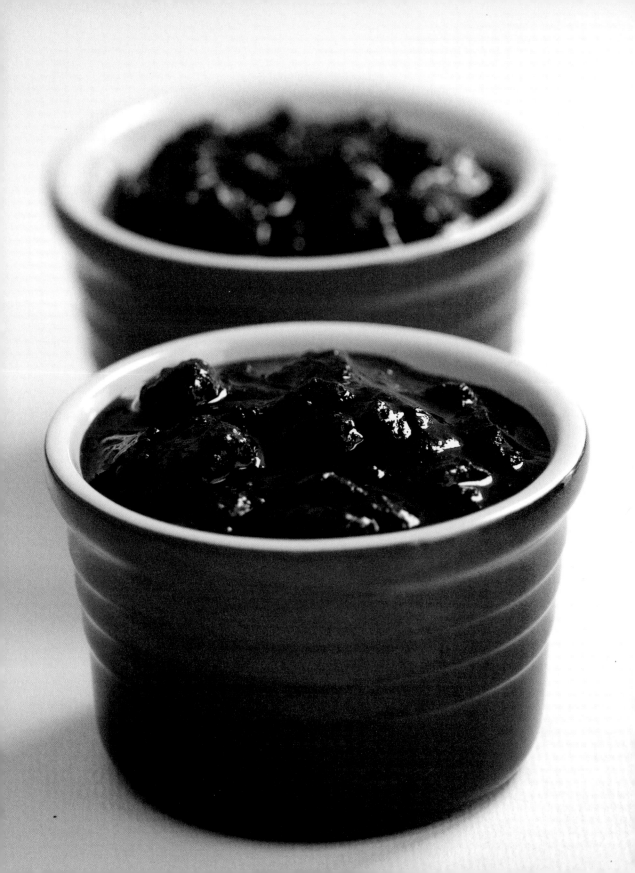

Whole Berry Sauce

Makes 3 cups

Y ou don't really need to doctor up berries too much. This is a very simple recipe that works with any sweet berry, fresh or frozen, and makes a luscious, thick sauce for filling your crepes or topping off your pancakes. The sweetness level will vary depending on the sweetness of your berries, so start with the 1/3 cup of sugar and add more if needed. I've used this recipe for raspberries, blueberries, marionberries, blackberries, and strawberries. If using strawberries, slice them in half and you're good to go.

4 cups berries, fresh or frozen

1/3 to 1/2 cup sugar

1 tablespoon arrowroot (cornstarch is okay, too)

2 tablespoons cold water

Combine all ingredients in a saucepan or saucier. Mix around to dissolve the arrowroot. Turn the heat up to medium. Stir the mixture often for about 15 minutes, until the sauce is thick and the berries are broken down a bit but still whole. If using frozen berries, the process will take a little longer. Let sit for at least 10 minutes before serving. I like this sauce best at room temperature.

☀ VARIATIONS ☀

CHERRY VANILLA BEAN

Use cherries (obviously) and scrape the **bean from 1 vanilla pod** into the sauce before cooking.

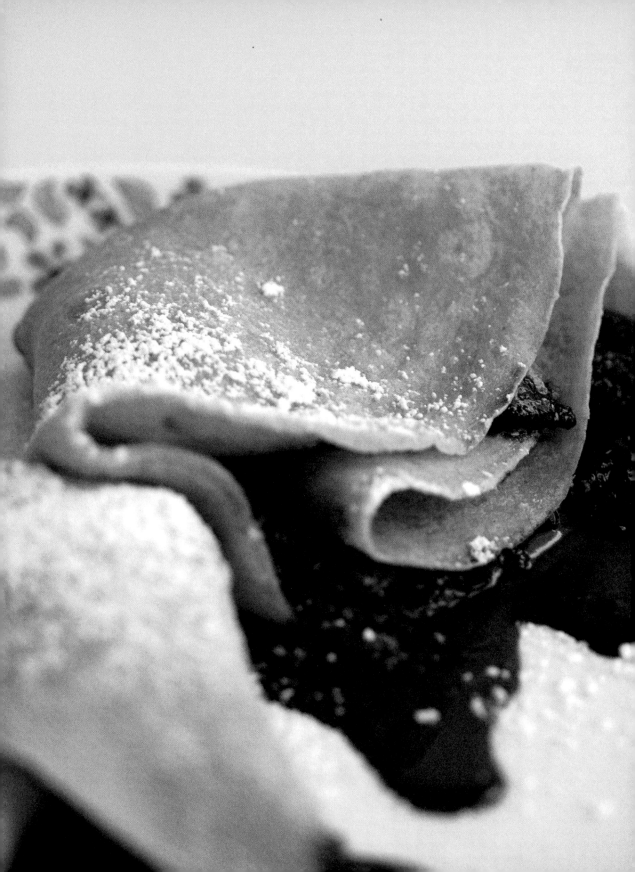

BLUEBERRY GINGER

Use blueberries, and when the sauce is done, mix in **1 tablespoon grated fresh ginger**.

RASPBERRY ORANGE

Use raspberries, **2 teaspoons orange zest**, and **½ cup fresh orange juice**; omit the water.

BLACKBERRY PASSION FRUIT

Use blackberries. When the sauce is done cooking add the **strained pulp of 2 passion fruits**.

STRAWBERRY ROSEWATER

Use strawberries sliced in half. When the sauce is done cooking add **2 tablespoons rosewater**.

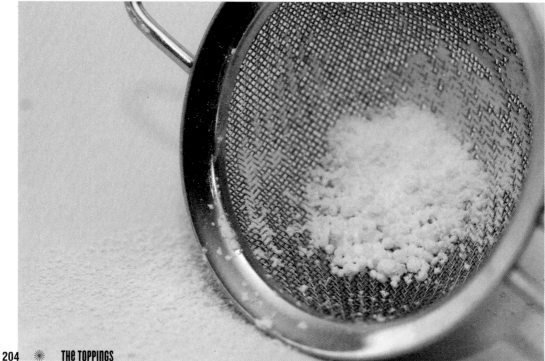

Brown Sugar
Peach Coulis

Makes about 3 cups

A coulis is simply a thick, pureed sauce, but having lots of words for "sauce" in your lexicon is sure to impress people at brunch soirees. If your peaches are really ripe then pureeing may not even be necessary; the peaches might just cook down all by themselves. Whatever the case, a blender isn't needed; you'll be able to mash the peaches with a fork to get the right consistency. This is great for the Old-Fashioned Chelsea Waffles (page 88)—the sauce fills all the crevices.

Combine all ingredients in a saucepan or saucier. Mix around to dissolve the arrowroot. Turn the heat up to medium. Stir the mixture often for about 15 minutes, until the sauce thickens and the peaches break down just a bit. Mash the peaches with a fork and cook for 5 more minutes. Serve when the sauce has stopped steaming.

4 cups peaches, peeled and roughly chopped

½ cup brown sugar

2 teaspoons arrowroot (cornstarch is okay, too)

2 teaspoons ground cinnamon

Caramelized Figs

Serves 4 to 6

Fresh figs are a treat in and of themselves, but place them under the broiler for a few minutes and they are nothing short of ambrosia. I love these on the Gingerbread Waffles (page 95), Pumpkin Pancakes (page 85), Pumpkin French Toast (page 101), or Banana Rabanada (page 102). They are best right out of the oven.

Approximately 1 pint fresh figs, any type

2 tablespoons sugar

Adjust broiler rack to be about 3 inches from the heat. Set the oven to broil. Slice the figs in half lengthwise.

Sprinkle sugar on a plate. Press each fig, cut side down, into the sugar to lightly coat. Lay figs cut side up in a single layer on a cookie sheet. Broil until the figs are bubbly and caramelized, 4 to 5 minutes. Serve immediately.

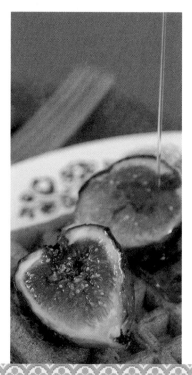

Baked Cinnamon Apples

Serves 4 to 6

This is a really simple topping, sort of like apple pie filling, and is very flexible. You can use any apples you like, but keep in mind that red generally cook faster than green and are a bit more sweet, so you may need to up the sugar by a few tablespoons if you're using an apple you know to be especially tart. I love these on top of the Raised Waffles (page 98), but honestly they can top off anything in the "Sweet" chapter really nicely.

2 pounds apples, peeled and sliced into a little less than ½-inch slices

¼ cup brown sugar

1 teaspoon ground cinnamon

Preheat the oven to 350°F.

Place the apple slices close together on a rimmed baking sheet lined with parchment paper. Sprinkle with the sugar and cinnamon. Cover the apples with tinfoil, leaving room for steam to escape, and bake for 15 minutes; then flip them and bake uncovered for about 5 minutes more, or until tender.

Chocolate Drizzle

Makes 1½ cups

Who couldn't use a little chocolate drizzled over ... everything? This rich sauce is very versatile and can make your entire brunch. See how yummy it looks on the Chocolate Beer Waffles (page 97). It's especially luscious when drizzled over strawberries and bananas. Try some of the variations below, and even the simplest brunch of pancakes will become something never to be forgotten.

In a saucepan with rounded sides, bring the milk to a boil. Bring the heat to low and add the chocolate chips, stirring constantly until the chips are dissolved. Add the vanilla, remove from the heat, and let cool. Serve when it has stopped steaming.

1 cup almond milk (or your preferred nondairy milk)
1 cup vegan chocolate chips
1 teaspoon pure vanilla extract

❊ VARIATIONS ❊

Any liqueur will fit right in here. Remove ¼ cup of the almond milk. Add ¼ **cup liqueur** when you add the vanilla. Some suggestions are coffee, hazelnut, coconut, almond, orange, or raspberry.

If you don't want to use liqueur but still want to try new flavors, here are a couple of ideas:

2 teaspoons of coffee extract
1 tablespoon orange zest

Sweet Cashew Cream

Makes about 1½ cups

Pureed cashews answer our prayers, turning into a smooth and creamy topping to drizzle over the fruit on our waffles and pancakes. You can use immediately if you would like a pourable cream, or refrigerate overnight if you would like a cream you need to spoon out.

½ cup raw cashew pieces

Water for submerging the cashews

1 cup almond milk

1 tablespoon agave nectar or pure maple syrup

½ teaspoon pure vanilla extract

In a small bowl, soak the cashew pieces in water for at least an hour and up to overnight. This softens them up and makes them the smoothest they can possibly be. Drain well.

Combine the drained cashews with the remaining ingredients in a blender or food processor. Puree until smooth, scraping down the sides with a spatula to make sure you get everything. Keep tightly sealed and refrigerated until ready to use. If refrigerated, it will firm up a bit in about an hour, and even more so in three hours.

TIP Cashews can be an expensive ingredient. To save some money, look for cashew pieces instead of whole cashews. Same great cashews and they come already chopped up, yet they're a few bucks cheaper. Go figure. We sure pulled one over on the cashew industry.

❋ VARIATIONS ❋

Add **1 teaspoon cinnamon** for cinnamon cashew cream.

Use **unsalted macadamia nuts** for macadamia cream.

Garden Herb Spread

Makes 2 cups

This is my favorite spread for bagels or crackers. It's creamy, herby, and perfect for that ferocious morning hunger when the scramble isn't quite ready yet.

In a food processor or blender, chop the cashews into coarse crumbs. Add the garlic and pulse to incorporate. Add the tofu, crumbling with your fingers as you drop it in. Blend until relatively smooth. Add everything else and pulse. You don't want the onion and herbs to completely puree; they should be chopped into small bits.

You can serve immediately, but I think this spread tastes best when it's chilled for at least a half hour.

½ cup raw cashew pieces

1 garlic clove, chopped

1 pound firm tofu, drained

2 tablespoons chopped fresh basil

2 tablespoons fresh thyme

1 tablespoon chopped fresh tarragon

2 tablespoons chopped fresh oregano

Fresh black pepper

2 tablespoons lemon juice (from 1 lemon)

¼ cup chopped red onion

¼ teaspoon salt

2 tablespoons nutritional yeast (optional)

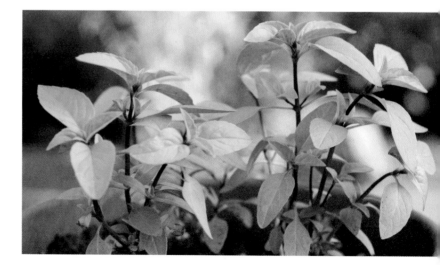

Cashew Sour Cream

Makes 1½ cups

This is a creamy condiment for Latin-inspired dishes. It doesn't taste like dairy sour cream, so don't expect that. Instead, expect something cool and tangy to temper your spicy foods.

Soak cashews in water for at least an hour and up to overnight.

Reserve ⅓ cup of water, and drain the cashews. Combine the cashews, the ⅓ cup of water, and the vinegar in a food processor. Blend until smooth, scraping down the sides with a spatula to make sure you get everything. Add onion and salt. Blend until smooth.

Refrigerate in a tightly sealed container for at least an hour. After an hour it will still be drippy, although still yummy. If you let the sour cream sit for 3 or more hours it firms up a lot.

1 cup raw cashew pieces

2 cups water

2 tablespoons red wine vinegar

2 tablespoons chopped yellow onion

¼ teaspoon salt

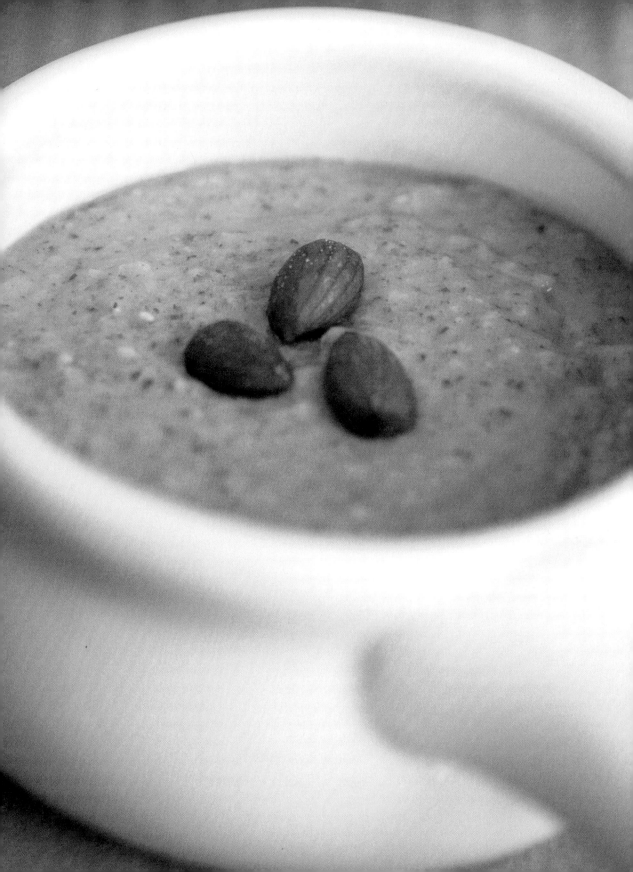

Smoked Almond Gravy

Makes 2 cups

I always sit on the couch and eat way too many smoked almonds. I was looking for a way to parlay that activity into brunch, and I found it in smoked almond gravy. This is one of those times where I think "Thank God I thought of this!" instead of "I wish I had thought of that!" Really rich, smoky gravy that is just perfect with biscuits. Not to mention it only uses a handful of ingredients and takes a handful of minutes. Smoked almonds are available in most supermarkets these days, and even at your local quick-e-mart.

2 garlic cloves

1 cup smoked almonds

1¼ cups water

2 tablespoons soy sauce

2 tablespoons cornstarch

Chop the garlic in a food processor or blender. Add the almonds and process into fine crumbs. Add the remaining ingredients and process until relatively smooth.

Transfer to a saucepot over medium heat. Stir often until thickened, about 5 minutes. That's it!

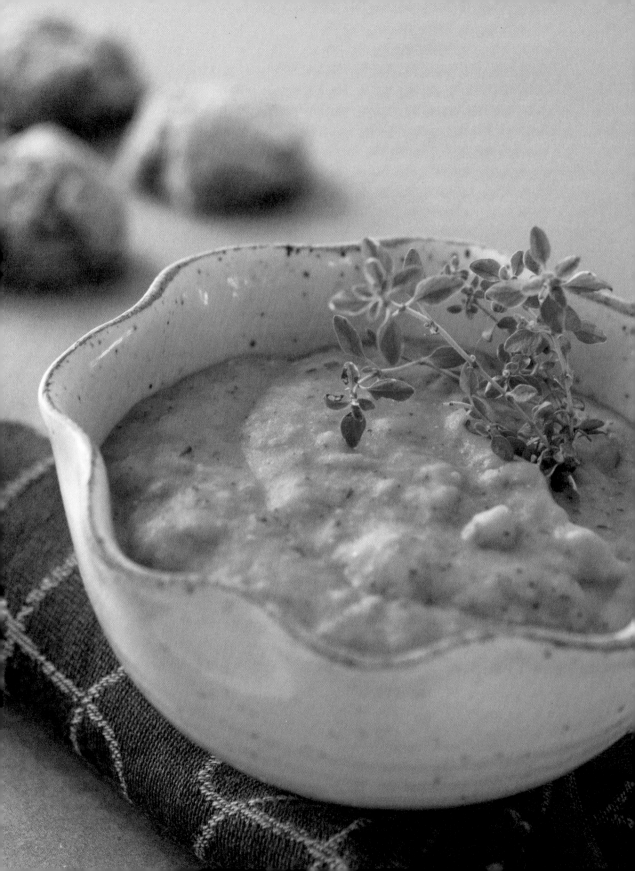

Navy Bean Gravy

Makes 2 cups

Most people seem to have a particular way they like their gravy. This one is of the thick, southern-style kinds that you serve on the side and is great for dipping your biscuit or potatoes in. It's also really wonderful with the Tempeh Sausage Pastry Puffs (page 129). Since everything is pureed, don't be too particular about how you chop the ingredients up. The thyme leaves don't have to be meticulously pulled from the stems; so long as the stems are tender enough just chop them up, too—that way everything comes together fast. An immersion blender comes in really handy here, but if you don't have one, a blender is just fine, too.

1 tablespoon olive oil

1 small onion, roughly chopped

3 garlic cloves, chopped

3 tablespoons fresh thyme, chopped

Several dashes fresh black pepper

1½ cups vegetable broth

⅓ cup flour

1 fifteen-ounce can navy beans, drained and rinsed

3 tablespoons soy sauce

¼ to ½ cup water

Salt, to taste (if needed)

Preheat a saucepan over medium-high heat. Sauté the onion and garlic in the oil for about 5 minutes. Add the thyme and black pepper (I like a lot of black pepper in this) and cook for about 3 minutes more. While that is cooking, stir the flour into the broth until dissolved.

If you have an immersion blender, then add the beans, broth mixture, and soy sauce to the saucepan. Blend immediately and lower the heat to medium. Stir the gravy often for about 10 minutes while it thickens.

If you are using a regular blender, add the beans, broth mixture, and soy sauce to the blender and blend until smooth. Transfer the onion and the other stuff from the pan to the blender. Puree again until no big chunks of onion are left. Add back to the pot and stir often over medium heat to thicken.

Once the gravy thickens, reduce the heat to low. Now you can decide exactly how thick you want it by adding splashes of water, anywhere from ¼ to ½ cup. Cook for about 20 more minutes to let the flavors deepen, stirring occasionally. Add water as necessary and taste for salt. Keep gravy covered and warm until ready to serve.

Mushroom Gravy

Makes about 6 cups

I admit that I could eat this by the bowlful, biscuits be damned. But if you have not achieved the level of vegan-ness that I have, you might want to serve it on stuff, like Basic Scrambled Tofu (page 19) or Tempeh Sausage Pastry Puffs (page 129) or on practically any brunch item that gets set in front of you. Except for French toast; don't do that.

Mix the flour into the broth until dissolved and set aside.

Preheat a large nonstick pan over medium heat. Sauté the onion in the oil for about 5 minutes, until translucent. Add the mushrooms and sauté for 5 more minutes, until the mushrooms are tender.

Add the garlic, thyme, sage, salt, and pepper. Sauté for another minute. Add the wine and turn the heat up to bring to a simmer. Let simmer for about a minute, then lower the heat and add the broth mixture. Stir constantly until thickened, about 5 minutes. If not serving the gravy immediately, gently reheat it when you are ready to serve.

2 cups vegetable broth

¼ cup flour (use ⅓ cup for a thicker gravy)

2 tablespoons olive oil

1 medium onion, thinly sliced into ½-inch-long pieces

10 ounces cremini mushrooms, thinly sliced (about 4 cups)

3 garlic cloves, minced

1 teaspoon thyme

½ teaspoon sage

¼ teaspoon salt

Several dashes fresh black pepper

¼ cup white cooking wine (or any nonsweet wine will do)

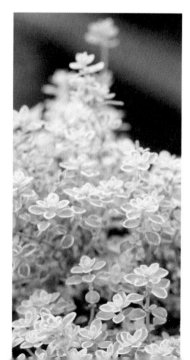

Cheesy Sauce

Makes about 3 cups

Who has the time or gumption to say "nutritional yeast" every time the magical pixie dust comes into conversation? My message boards have come up with a convenient shorthand: nooch. This is the nooch sauce that I use whenever I need a melty, cheesy topping for a meal.

Combine the broth and flour in a measuring cup and whisk with a fork until the flour is dissolved (a couple of lumps are okay).

Preheat a small saucepan over medium-low heat. Add the oil and garlic and gently cook the garlic for about 2 minutes, stirring often and being careful not to burn the garlic.

Add the thyme, salt, and pepper and cook for about 15 seconds. Add the broth mixture, turmeric, and nutritional yeast and bring the heat up to medium. Use a whisk to stir pretty constantly. It should start bubbling and thickening in about 3 minutes; if it doesn't then turn the heat a bit higher.

Once bubbling and thickening, stir the sauce for about 2 more minutes. Add the lemon juice and mustard. It should resemble a thick, melty cheese. Taste for salt (you may need more depending on how salty your vegetable broth is), turn the heat off, and cover to keep warm until ready to use. The top might set a bit while it sits, but you can just stir it and it will be fine. Serve warm.

2 cups vegetable broth (or water)

¼ cup all-purpose flour

1 tablespoon olive oil

3 garlic cloves, minced

A pinch dried thyme (crumbled in your fingers)

¼ teaspoon salt

A few dashes fresh black pepper

⅛ teaspoon turmeric

¾ cup nutritional yeast

1 tablespoon fresh lemon juice

1 teaspoon yellow prepared mustard

Hollandaise Sauce

Makes 2 cups

This is for the Tofu Benny (page 67), but it's also wonderful as a sauce on the side. Pour it on your home fries, your scrambled tofu, your roommate's head. ...

In a saucier or small sauce pot, sauté the shallot in oil for about 3 minutes over medium heat. In the meantime, mix the milk with the arrowroot in a measuring cup. Stir until the arrowroot is mostly dissolved and set aside.

Add the white wine and vinegar to the shallots. Turn the heat all the way up and bring to a boil. Cook for about 5 minutes, until the liquid has reduced to about 2 tablespoons. While it's reducing, you can add the turmeric and broth powder to the milk mixture.

Once the liquid has reduced, add the milk mixture to the pan and lower the heat to medium. Whisk pretty consistently for 5 to 7 minutes, until the sauce thickens. I'll stress this point, because if you don't whisk it will be lumpy. So whisk! Once sauce is thickened, mix in the nutritional yeast, lemon juice, and salt. It tastes best if you let it cool for at least 20 minutes. The milk taste will mellow out and disappear and the flavors will all marry, so do cover and let it sit for a bit. If it cools too much, that's fine, just gently reheat. But it tastes best just slightly warmer than room temperature.

2 tablespoons olive oil

¼ cup minced shallots (one shallot)

1½ cups unsweetened almond milk (or soy milk)

2 tablespoons plus 1 teaspoon arrowroot

¼ cup white wine

3 tablespoons white wine vinegar

¼ teaspoon turmeric

2 tablespoons vegetable broth powder

2 tablespoons nutritional yeast

1 tablespoon fresh lemon juice

¼ teaspoon salt

Cashew Ricotta

Makes 2 cups

This ricotta is originally from *Veganomicon*, but it is outstanding in the omelet filled with Roasted Tomatoes, Ricotta, and Basil (page 15), so here is the recipe again, for your convenience.

In a food processor, blend together the cashews, lemon juice, olive oil, and garlic until a thick creamy paste forms. Add the crumbled tofu to the food processor, working in two or more batches if necessary, until the mixture is thick and well blended. Blend in the basil and add salt, to taste.

½ cup raw cashew pieces (approximately 4 ounces)

¼ cup fresh lemon juice

2 tablespoons olive oil

2 cloves fresh or roasted garlic

1 pound firm tofu, drained and crumbled

1½ teaspoons dried basil

1½ teaspoons salt

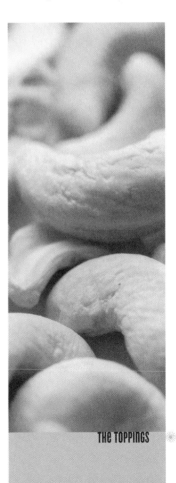

Miso Tahini Sauce

Makes 1 cup

his sauce is a really simple-to-throw-together way to enjoy omelets; I especially love it with the Grilled Marinated Asparagus filling (page 15).

½ cup tahini

½ cup water

1 tablespoon miso

1 teaspoon balsamic vinegar

Combine everything in a blender and go to town. Blend until thoroughly combined.

Guacamole

Serves 6

Everyone has their guacamole preference and is extremely offended if anyone tries to tell them another way to make it. This is how I like my guac! If you have another preference, by all means, use it.

Scoop avocado out into a medium-size mixing bowl. Use a strong fork to mix in the rest of the ingredients. Really squish the onion and tomato in there, almost like you are pulverizing it with the fork. I love the flavor that the tomato juice gives to the guac. Keep tightly sealed and refrigerated until ready to use and don't make any earlier than an hour before you plan on serving. Place an avocado pit in the guac to help keep it from discoloring.

2 ripe avocados

¼ cup finely chopped red onion

1 plum tomato, finely chopped

2 tablespoons finely chopped cilantro

Juice from 1 lime

½ teaspoon salt, or to taste

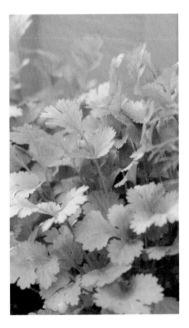

The Drinks

Just When You
Thought You Knew
How to Make a Smoothie

Bloody Moskowitz

Makes 1 drink

There's nothing like a tangy, zesty tomato juice to get you going in the morning. And that shot of vodka can't hurt either! But truth be told, I actually drink these virgin. I have two secret ingredients that make these "Mary's" into Moskowitz's. One is pickle juice and the other is liquid smoke. And if that don't sound right to you, I promise after three or four of these it will begin to.

Fill a drink shaker with ice and add all the ingredients except for the pepper, celery stalk, and lemon. Give her a good shake. Fill a big glass with ice and grind a few dashes of fresh pepper on top of the ice. Strain the drink into the glass, stick in the celery stalk, and pop on the lemon wedge. Sprinkle with a little Kosher salt. Serve with straws.

1½ ounces vodka

¾ cup tomato vegetable juice

2 tablespoons pickle juice

2 teaspoons grated horseradish

Juice of ½ lemon

A dash of liquid smoke

1 teaspoon hot sauce

Fresh black pepper

Stalk of celery for garnish

Lemon wedges for garnish

Kosher salt for garnish

Pink Grapefruit Mimosas

Tired of those orange mimosas? This little twist will give you a great reason to pop the cork. I'm not going to give you yield quantities; you should just be able to eyeball these babies.

3 parts fresh ruby red grapefruit juice

1 part agave nectar

3 parts champagne

Mix the grapefruit juice with the agave. Pour in the champagne. That's it!

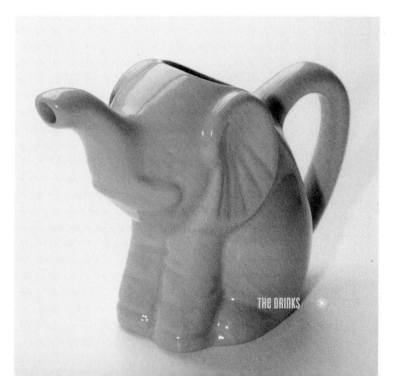

Smoothies Supreme

Makes 4 smoothies

I made a vow to myself that I would never put a smoothie recipe in a book, but I need to set the record straight. Ice does not belong in a smoothie! Because ice is made of water (did you know that?), all it does is water down the flavor of your smoothie. And for the love of all that is good and holy, can we keep the kale out of the smoothie, people? Just put it on your plate, the way God intended. The secret to Smoothies Supreme is frozen fruit and a little pineapple juice. Now you're on the road to opening a smoothie joint in the mall. You're welcome.

Add everything to a blender and puree away. Serve in a big glass with a straw and a few extra berries on top for cuteness.

2 cups frozen berries (my favorite combo is blueberry and raspberry)

2 frozen bananas

1 cup nondairy milk

1 cup pineapple juice

TIP When bananas are just beginning to brown, peel them, break them in half, store in plastic bags, and freeze. Always have them at the ready for when a smoothie moment strikes.

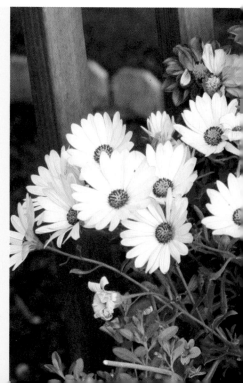

Mango Lassi

Makes 4 drinks

The sweetness of mangoes and the sourness of yogurt will make you suck this through the straw at breakneck speed. A little cardamom adds some spice to this traditional Northern Indian drink. Use frozen mangoes for the best, thickest texture, but I've been known to just puree the mangoes fresh when I didn't get a chance to prepare ahead.

Add everything to a blender except for the lime wedges. Puree until smooth. Serve in a big glass with a straw and garnish with lime wedges.

2 mangoes, peeled, cubed, and
    frozen (about 3 cups)

1 cup nondairy milk

1 container nondairy yogurt
    (preferably coconut)

2 to 3 tablespoons agave nectar

¼ teaspoon ground cardamom

Lime wedges for garnish

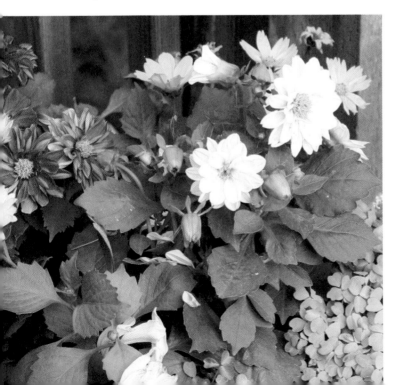

Black-and-White Le Cremes

Makes 1 drink

Chocolate and vanilla living together in harmony? Unheard of! As a child in NYC these were heaven in a luncheonette to me. Chocolate and vanilla syrup, fizzy seltzer, and creamy almond milk: the perfect soft drink. Even though egg creams don't have any actual egg in them these days, I still changed the name because that's what vegans do. Keep all ingredients very cold and do not under any circumstances serve these over ice; that is sacrilegious. Serve in the biggest glass you've got.

Pour milk and seltzer into a large glass. Add the syrups and use a long spoon to stir. It's a nice touch to keep the spoon in the glass when you serve the drink. Drink with a straw.

1 cup almond milk

1 cup seltzer

1½ tablespoons chocolate syrup

1½ tablespoons vanilla syrup

Acknowledgments

Like crazy, I thank the following:

Justin Field for cleaning the kitchen no matter how much of a mess I made (and you have no idea what I am capable of), setting up the photo shoots, keeping the cat hair out of the quiches and eating as much scrambled tofu as I could throw his way.

My photo assistants and stylists:

Jess Denoto, for holding that lighting thing like a pro and fearlessly making scones.

Kimmy Kokonut for making cinnamon rolls when I thought I could never roll anything ever again.

Kevin Schmidt for making waffles and aiming the camera at things.

Terry Hope Romero, who was with me in spirit, even if in reality she was in Queens.

Josh Hooten, Michelle Schweggers, and Ruby Bird Hooten for coming over and eating bagels. Who else would have eaten the bagels?!

Chad Miller and Emiko Badillo, for constantly dissing brunch at every turn, making me that much more determined to prove myself. And for providing me with vital wheat gluten.

Mom, because I have to thank you in every book.

The Brown Klan: Mish, Aaron, Max and baby Norah for being adorable, the lot of you.

Jenny Brown at Woodstock Farm Sanctuary and Sarah Downs at Farm Sanctuary CA for doing such great work with such great animals and giving me more and more reasons to provide vegan alternatives to the standard American breakfast.

Katie, Christine, Jane, Georgia, and Wesley at Perseus for helping to make the book as beautiful as a berry muffin.

Brunch truly is about community and my testers proved that. This cookbook would not have been possible had they not given their feedback, let me know what worked and what didn't and even fixed my typos. I love you guys! I hope you know that whenever you are in town I will whip up some scramble for you.

Lisa "pandacookie" Coulson — Thumbs up to muffins

Bahar "bazu" Zaker — Brakes for beer battered tofu

Abby "Tootsie" Wohl — Frittata fatale

Carrie Lynn "supercarrot" Morse — Cherry sage sausages for the win

Paul "ijustdiedinside" Gross — Fights evil with butterscotch

Katie "badmouth" Hubbard — Runs game on tofu

Erica "catsgalore" Johnson — Making tempeh bacon back in

Tami "AsstroGirl" Noyes — Takes tempeh hostage

Thalia "veganmd" C. Palmer — Gives good omelet

Liz Bujack & Mike Crooker — Private Benedict

Amanda "esme" Sacco — bESt tEstEr eVeRZ

Carla "Queen V" Kelly — Quiche for a day

Lucy "superherogirl" Allbaugh — Dreams of fennel rissoto (but totally innocently)

Allicia "no Xs" Cormier

Dayna "SeitanSaidDance" Rozental — Heart of artichoke

Rose "bike rides and high 5s" Hermalin — Fork this shiitake

Eryn "seitanicverses" Hiscock — Agave slave

John Plummer — Stuck in the barley malt

Jessica L. DeNoto — Sconed

Kristen Blackmore

Kim "vit" Carpenter (soon to be Lahn) — The Esme of the brunch book

Fred "phatty" Lahn — Partner in cremini

Becca "bex" Bennett — You gonna eat that?

Shanell Dawn Williams – Tempehstress

Julie Farson — Maple mama

Jessica Bauer — Flapjack of all trades

Megan "sugarcookie" Duke — Coockoo for Cocoa Muffins

Melisser "And Strummer" Elliot

Molly "The Veganatrix" Tanzer

Liz "EFCliz" Wyman — All praise the Pierogi!!

Evan "rayray" Maxwell William Mcgraw — Peanut butter

Michele "t-tat" Thompson-Brayton — Gives a crepe

Zac "Dan" Watts — Beer battered

Jeff "jeff" Press — Linguist

Angela White

Amy Sims

Jane Ott

Index

Flour
chickpea flour, 3–4, 13, 126
gluten-free recipes and, 82, 126
whole wheat flour recipes, 104–105, 186–187
See also Buckwheat flour; Spelt flour
Food Fight! Vegan Grocery, 18, 73
Freezing
bananas, 226
waffles, 89
French toast
Banana Rabanada (Brazilian French Toast), 102–103, 206
Pumpkin French Toast, 100–101, 206
tips on, 101
Fresh Herb Roasted Potatoes, 113
Fresh Mango Muffins, 166
Fried Plantains, 135, 151
Frittata
about, 33
Curried Cauliflower Frittata, 38–39, 125
Shiitake Dill Frittata, 37
Swiss Chard Frittata, 34–36

Garden Herb Spread, 67, 193, 194, 210
Garlic
Garlic Roasted Potatoes, 113
Jalapeño Garlic Grits, 127
Ginger
Blueberry Ginger Sauce, 204
Blueberry Ginger Spelt Muffins, 154–155
Ginger Cranberry Sauce, 84–85, 200–201
Gingerbread Waffles, 94–95, 206

Simple Stuffed Artichokes with Ginger and Chervil, 146–147
tips on, 155
Gluten-free recipes
Gluten-Free Buckwheat Pancakes, 82
Samosa Mashed Potato Pancakes, 126
Grapefruit, Pink Grapefruit Mimosas, 225
Gravy
Mushroom Gravy, 216
Navy Bean Gravy, 214–215
Red Wine Tarragon Mushroom Gravy, 63
Smoked Almond Gravy, 212–213
Greens
Sautéed Collards and Sausages, 142–143
Sesame Scrambled Tofu and Greens with Yams, 30
Grilled Marinated Asparagus omelet filling, 15, 220
Grilled Pineapple Salsa, 73–75, 76, 118, 151
Grits
Jalapeño Garlic Grits, 127
polenta vs., 127
tips on, 127
Guacamole, 16, 17, 32, 33, 51, 61, 135, 221

Hash Browns, Individual, 114–115
Hasson, Julie, 137
Herb (Fresh) Roasted Potatoes, 113
Herb spread, Garden Herb Spread, 67, 193, 194, 210
Herbed Whole Wheat Drop Biscuits, 186–187
Hollandaise Sauce, 66–68, 218
Hominy, 127

Individual Hash Browns, 114–115
Ingredient sources
Food Fight! Vegan Grocery, 18, 73
Penzeys Spices, 130
Ingredient supplies, 3–5
Injera bread, 77
Italian Feast Sausages, 140

Jalapeños
Cornbread Biscuits with, 192
Jalapeño Garlic Grits, 127
Jam Swirl Coffee Cake, 175

Kala namak (black salt), 4, 67

Ladles, 71, 106–107
Lavender, 182
Leeks, Mushroom, Leek, and White Bean Pie, 45–46
Lemon pepper
about, 130
Lemon Pepper Roasted Potatoes, 113
Lemon Pepper Tofu, 131
Lemons
Lemon Cashew-Stuffed Crepes with Whole Berry Sauce, 104, 108–109
Lemon Poppy Seed Muffins, 158–159
Liqueur and Chocolate Drizzle, 208
Liquid smoke, 5

Macadamia Cream, 209
Mangoes
Fresh Mango Muffins, 166
Mango Lassi, 227
Toasted Coconut and Mango Muffins, 164–166
Marionberries, 182
Matzoh Brie, 53
Menu planning, 7